Perioperative Temperature Management

Perioperative Temperature Management

Anselm Bräuer

Department of Anaesthesiology, University of Göttingen, Germany

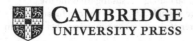

CAMBRIDGE
UNIVERSITY PRESS

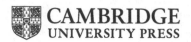

Shaftesbury Road, Cambridge CB2 8EA, United Kingdom

One Liberty Plaza, 20th Floor, New York, NY 10006, USA

477 Williamstown Road, Port Melbourne, VIC 3207, Australia

314–321, 3rd Floor, Plot 3, Splendor Forum, Jasola District Centre, New Delhi – 110025, India

103 Penang Road, #05–06/07, Visioncrest Commercial, Singapore 238467

Cambridge University Press is part of Cambridge University Press & Assessment, a department of the University of Cambridge.

We share the University's mission to contribute to society through the pursuit of education, learning and research at the highest international levels of excellence.

www.cambridge.org
Information on this title: www.cambridge.org/9781107535770

DOI: 10.1017/9781316335963

First published 2017

A catalogue record for this publication is available from the British Library

Library of Congress Cataloging-in-Publication data
Names: Bräuer, Anselm, 1965- author.
Title: Perioperative temperature management / Anselm Bräuer.
Description: Cambridge, United Kingdom ; New York, NY : Cambridge
University Press, 2017. | Includes bibliographical references and index.
Identifiers: LCCN 2017000020 | ISBN 9781107535770 (pbk. : alk. paper)
Subjects: | MESH: Anesthesia–adverse effects | Hypothermia–prevention
& control | Perioperative Care–methods | Body Temperature–physiology
Classification: LCC RM863 | NLM WO 245 | DDC 615.8/329–dc23
LC record available at https://lccn.loc.gov/2017000020

ISBN   978-1-107-53577-0   Paperback

Contents

Preface   vii

SECTION 1 Introduction

1. History of perioperative
   hypothermia   1

2. Physiology of heat and cold
   sensation   9

3. Physiology of thermoregulation   17

4. Physiology of heat gain and
   heat loss   26

SECTION 2 Changes induced by anaesthesia and surgery

5. Influence of preanaesthetic core
   temperature and premedication   33

6. Influence of transportation to the
   operating room and preparation for
   surgery   42

7. Influence of general
   anaesthesia   44

8. Influence of regional
   anaesthesia   59

9. Influence of regional anaesthesia
   and sedation   65

10. Influence of epidural anaesthesia
    and general anaesthesia   68

11. Influence of the surgical
    environment and surgery   71

SECTION 3 Adverse effects of perioperative hypothermia

12. Incidence of perioperative
    hypothermia   75

13. Influence on pharmacokinetics and
    pharmacodynamics   78

14. Influence on coagulation and
    blood loss   85

15. Feeling cold and shivering   91

16. Postoperative pain, pulmonary
    complications and length of
    stay in the postanaesthetic
    care unit   96

17. Cardiovascular consequences   98

18. Influence on wound healing and
    infections   103

19. Postoperative protein catabolism,
    length of stay, costs and
    mortality   108

SECTION 4 Measurement of core temperature

20. Equipment to measure core
    temperature   111

21. Measurement of core
    temperature   115

SECTION 5 Equipment and methods to keep patients warm

22. **Forced-air warmers**   128

23. **Conductive warmers**   143

24. **Infusion warmers**   152

25. **Warming of irrigation fluids**   158

26. **Insulation**   159

27. **Radiative warmers**   162

28. **Airway heating and humidification**   164

29. **Oesophageal warmers, negative-pressure warmers and endovascular warming catheters**   165

30. **Augmentation of heat production by amino acids or fructose**   167

SECTION 6 Perioperative temperature management

31. **Modern perioperative temperature management**   168

32. **Prewarming**   170

33. **Warming therapy during anaesthesia**   178

34. **Postoperative therapy**   184

References   187

Index   209

Preface

This book is designed for anaesthesiologists, anaesthesia nurses and surgeons who need more than a basic knowledge about perioperative temperature management. The book explains basic thermal physiology, the changes that are induced by anaesthesia and surgery, and then lists all the adverse outcomes that are associated with perioperative hypothermia. In the following sections all the necessary relevant information is given to prevent perioperative hypothermia, as well as some practical tips and tricks. I hope that the book can thereby offer some help in implementing temperature management more into daily practice and thereby help to protect more patients from the adverse outcomes that are associated with perioperative hypothermia.

Chapter

1

History of perioperative hypothermia

Perioperative hypothermia is one of the oldest known side effects of general anaesthesia and is still a very common problem today.

First description of perioperative hypothermia

Perioperative hypothermia was first described by Ernst von Bibra and Emil Harlass in Erlangen (Germany) in the book *Die Wirkung des Schwefeläthers in chemischer und physiologischer Beziehung* (Fig. 1.1) in the year 1847, only 1 year after the first successful general anaesthesia was performed by Thomas Green Morton in Boston.

In this book von Bibra and Harness describe results from human and animal experiments with sulfuric ether. The authors describe that the pharyngeal temperature of a rabbit had fallen to 24.5 °Réaumur under ether anaesthesia, which corresponds to a temperature of 30.6 °C. In contrast, a normal heathy rabbit had a pharyngeal temperature of 31.5 °Réaumur (= 39.4 °C). However, these results of a drop in core temperature under anaesthesia did not get very much attention as there were many more important problems associated with anaesthesia at that time.

Measurement of core temperature and definition of hypothermia

In the middle of the nineteenth century Carl Reinhold August Wunderlich introduced thermometry and temperature charts into hospitals and declared thermometry imperative in ill patients.

In 1868 Wunderlich published the book *Das Verhalten der Eigenwärme in Krankheiten*, in which he analysed over 1 million axillary temperature recordings from some 25 000 patients. He identified 37.0 °C as the mean temperature of healthy adults and declared that the normal temperature range extends from 36.25 °C to 37.5 °C.

A core temperature below 36 °C was only found in very severe illness. In his opinion a core temperature below 36.25 °C should only be considered to be normal under special circumstances. This may be the first scientific definition of hypothermia.

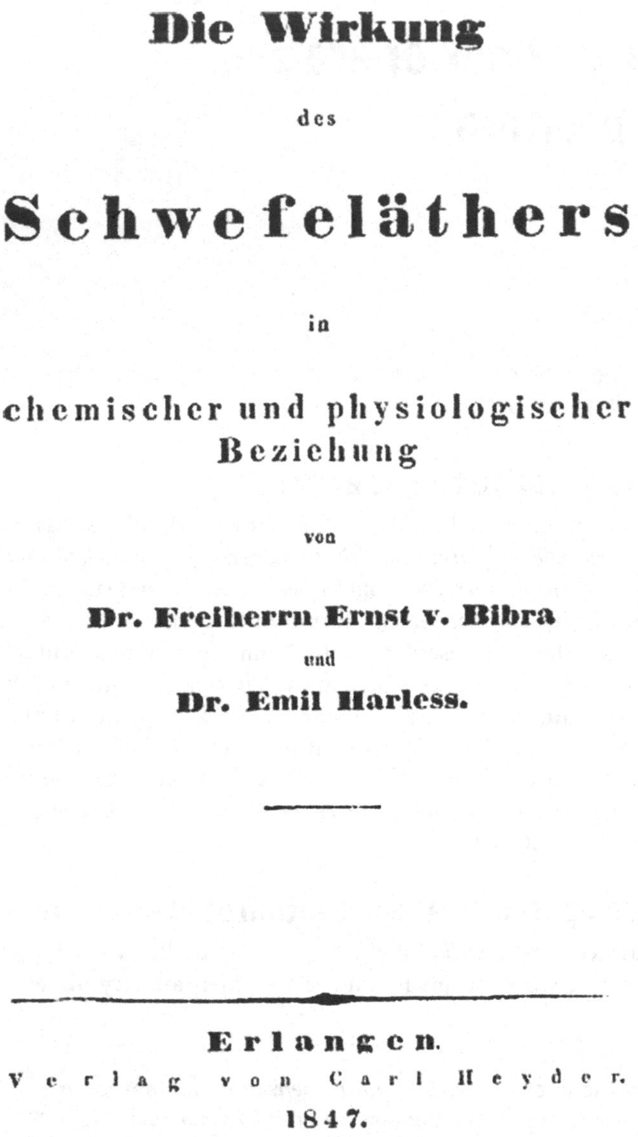

Die Wirkung

des

Schwefeläthers

in

chemischer und physiologischer Beziehung

von

Dr. Freiherrn Ernst v. Bibra

und

Dr. Emil Harless.

Erlangen.

Verlag von Carl Heyder.

1847.

Fig. 1.1 Cover of the book *Die Wirkung des Schwefeläthers in chemischer und physiologischer Beziehung* by von Bibra and Harness. (Reproduced from: Von Hintzenstern U, Petermann H and Schwarz W. Frühe Erlanger Beiträge zur Theorie und Praxis der Äther- und Chloroformnarkose. Teil 2. Die tierexperimentellen Untersuchungen von Ernst von Bibra und Emil Harless. Anaesthesist 2001; **50**: 869–880 [1] with kind permission of Springer Science and Business Media.)

First descriptions of adverse effects of perioperative hypothermia and first measures against hypothermia

In 1880, von Kappeler described a decrease in body temperature in 20 surgical patients. In 1881, the gynaecologist Emil Schwarz from Halle in Germany recommended warming infusion fluids to 38–40 °C to prevent cooling of the body. In 1907 Döderlein and König described an association between postoperative pneumonia and perioperative hypothermia. They recommended warmed operating tables, which could reduce pneumonia rates that ranged between 7.5 to 10.2% down to 3.6 to 2.1%. In the same year the surgeon Christian Heinrich Braun from Göttingen in Germany tried to prevent hypothermia

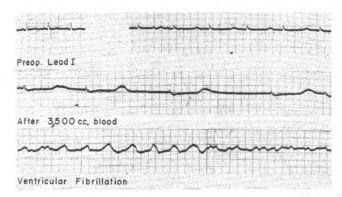

Fig. 1.2 Original electrocardiogram (ECG) recording in a patient with massive transfusion of cold blood. (Reproduced from: Howland WS, Boyan CP, Schweizer O. Ventricular fibrillation during massive blood replacement. Am J Surg 1956; **92**: 356–360 [2] with permission of Elsevier.)

during surgery by placing the patients on warm water cushions and by covering them with warm towels.

Severe perioperative hypothermia as a cause of death during massive transfusions

In 1956, Howland *et al.* [2] described nine cases of ventricular fibrillation during abdominal operations that were associated with rapid massive transfusion of cold blood. They speculated that one of the important pathophysiological factors was that cold blood was delivered directly to the heart, thereby causing cooling of the myocardium and leading to cardiac arrhythmias and ventricular fibrillation (Fig. 1.2).

In a subsequent prospective study [3] an oesophageal temperature probe was used to measure core temperature as close to the heart as possible during a massive transfusion of blood. In the first patient, the core temperature only dropped from 37 °C to 36 °C during the first 3000 ml of blood transfusion. During the following 120 minutes the patient needed 18 000 ml of cold bank blood at an average rate of 150 ml min^{-1}. During this period the oesophageal temperature decreased steadily. At 31 °C the first ventricular extrasystoles appeared and at 29 °C there was a marked prolongation of the ST-interval followed by bradycardia and ventricular extrasystoles. All cardiac function ceased at 27.5 °C although the estimated blood loss had been completely replaced.

In another patient, asystole appeared at a core temperature of 32 °C after transfusion of 6 600 ml of cold blood. Several other patients developed severe hypothermia during massive transfusions with core temperatures of about 30 to 32 °C. Because of these observations the authors decided to transfuse warm blood after the third unit of banked blood had been administered. Therefore they used a blood warmer consisting of more than 7 meters of sterile plastic tubing placed in a 20 l water bath with a bath thermometer (Fig. 1.3). The temperature of this water bath was regulated by adding warm or cold water.

With this blood warmer subsequent patients remained relatively warm, well above 35 °C, during massive transfusions and none of them developed arrhythmia or cardiac arrest.

A few years later Churchill-Davidson stated that hypothermia was the most important problem in massive blood transfusions. Even if the blood has been partially warmed, a massive transfusion can reduce the body temperature to a dangerously low level [4].

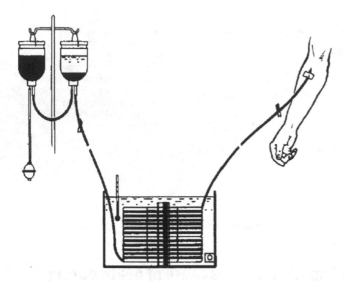

Fig. 1.3 Schematic drawing of the blood warmer. (Reproduced from: Boyan CP and Howland WS. Blood temperature: A critical factor in massive transfusion. Anesthesiology 1961; **22**: 559–563 [3] with kind permission of Wolters Kluwer Health.)

Severe perioperative hypothermia in paediatric anaesthesia

Another field where perioperative hypothermia was associated with severe problems was the emerging field of paediatric surgery and anaesthesia. In 1957, France [5] described relevant drops in core temperature down to 28.6 °C in newborns. The hypothermic children were drowsy with a slow respiration and rewarming took several hours. Hacket and Crosby [6] found that postoperative feeding problems in infants were associated with a fall in the core temperature below 36.1 °C. In 1962, Farman described an association of severe perioperative hypothermia with perioperative death in babies [7]. Nine of 67 babies undergoing surgery died within the first 24 hours; six of them suffered from hypothermia, with temperatures below 36.1 °C.

> The major cause of death in the hypothermic babies was respiratory depression [7].

In this article, Farman also searched for risk factors for perioperative hypothermia. He discussed an association with:

- Severity of illness
- Effect of low body weight
- Young age
- Anaesthetic drugs
- Muscle relaxants
- Long operations
- Air conditioning.

Harrison *et al.* [8] added:

- Intra-abdominal or intrathoracic procedures
- Low initial core temperature
- Transfusion of cold blood.

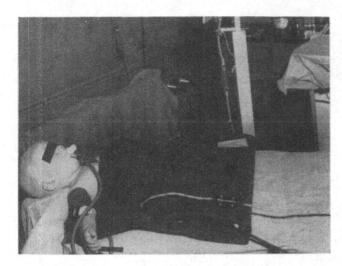

Fig. 1.4 Electrical heating blanket to maintain normothermia for a craniotomy in an infant. (Reproduced from: Bering EA Jr, Matson DD. A technique for the prevention of severe hypothermia during surgery of infants. Ann Surg 1953; **137**: 407–409 [11] with kind permission of Wolters Kluwer Health.)

First warming devices against perioperative hypothermia

Severe hypothermia in children and the dramatic observations of deaths due to perioperative hypothermia led to the development of several warming devices. In addition to blood and fluid warming devices [9, 10] heating mattresses were developed. In 1953, Bering and Matson [11] successfully used an electrical heating blanket to maintain normothermia during neurosurgical operations in infants (Fig. 1.4). The blanket measured about 60 × 100 cm overall, but was designed to be folded in the middle and closed with snap buttons on two sides. This allowed its use as a bottom or top blanket or to cover the patient on all sides. The temperature of this electrical heating mattress was controlled by a ten-step regulator switch and had a maximum temperature of slightly over 43 °C. The authors were convinced that the early postoperative recovery of infants undergoing all types of major neurosurgical procedure was strikingly accelerated when severe hypothermia had been obviated (Fig. 1.5).

In 1962, Calvert [12] described the use of a circulating water mattress in babies (Fig. 1.6). This rubber mattress was placed on the operating table and warm water from the hot and cold supply of the theatre continually circulated through the mattress. The temperature was regulated by varying the proportions of hot and cold water flowing through the mattress using a thermostatic mixing valve (Fig. 1.7).

They observed that the infants in their control group had a difference between preoperative and postoperative core temperature of 2.4 °C, whereas the infants that were warmed with the water mattress had an overall drop in core temperature of only 0.3 °C.

In 1973, Lewis et al. [13] described the first forced-air warming system for infants and could prove the efficacy of the system (Figs. 1.8 and 1.9).

With all these measures it was possible to prevent severe hypothermia. However, in the early 1980s as many as 50 to 80% of all patients still arrived hypothermic in the recovery room [14]. At that time mild perioperative hypothermia was considered a normal consequence of surgery, and not thought to be especially harmful. The only serious complication was thought to be the common postoperative shivering, because it

A

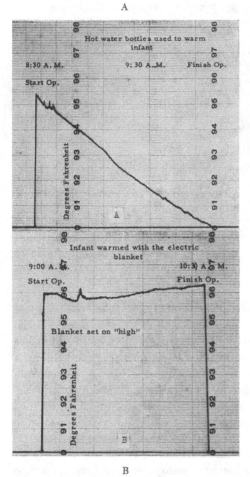

B

Fig. 1.5 Original recording of the rectal temperature of two infants during hydrocephalus operations. The first infant was warmed with hot water bottles as usual and the operation ended with a core temperature of 90 °F = 32.2 °C, whereas the second infant was warmed with the electrical heating blanket and the operation ended at a core temperature of 96.4 °F = 35.8 °C. (Reproduced from: Bering EA Jr, Matson DD. A technic for the prevention of severe hypothermia during surgery of infants. Ann Surg 1953; **137**: 407–409 [11] with kind permission of Wolters Kluwer Health.)

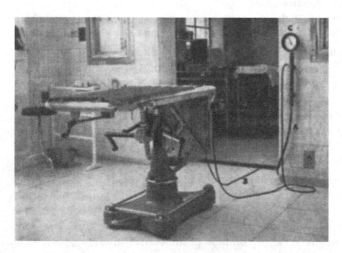

Fig. 1.6 The hot water mattress in position on the table. (Reproduced from: Calvert DG. Inadvertent hypothermia in paediatric surgery and a method for its prevention. Anaesthesia 1962; **17**: 29–45 [12] (Copyright by John Wiley and Sons) with kind permission of John Wiley and Sons.)

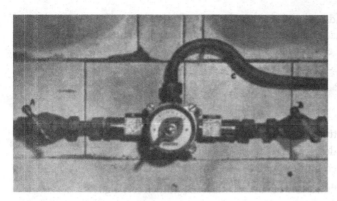

Fig. 1.7 The mixing valve controlling the water temperature in the mattress. (Reproduced from: Calvert DG. Inadvertent hypothermia in paediatric surgery and a method for its prevention. Anaesthesia 1962; **17**: 29–45 [12] (Copyright by John Wiley and Sons) with kind permission of John Wiley and Sons.)

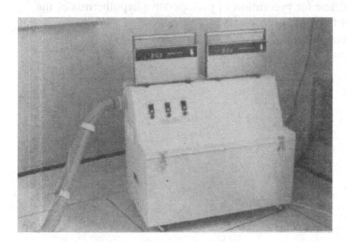

Fig. 1.8 The controller of the forced-air warmer used by Lewis. (Reproduced from: Lewis RB, Shaw A, Etchells AH. Contact mattress to prevent heat loss in neonatal and paediatric surgery. Br J Anaesth 1973; **45**: 919–922 [13] with kind permission of Oxford University Press.)

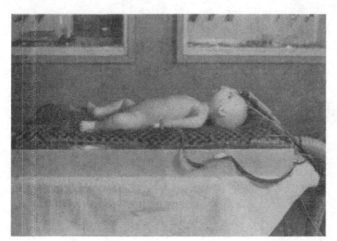

Fig. 1.9 The underbody forced-air warmer blanket used by Lewis. (Reproduced from: Lewis RB, Shaw A, Etchells AH. Contact mattress to prevent heat loss in neonatal and paediatric surgery. Br J Anaesth 1973; **45**: 919–922 [13] with kind permission of Oxford University Press.)

can increase oxygen demand and oxygen uptake [15]. Perioperative hypothermia was assumed to be caused by anaesthetics that switch off all thermoregulatory defences and by excessive heat loss to the environment [16].

In the next 20 years, new concepts for intraoperative thermoregulation were described and the adverse side effects of mild perioperative hypothermia were discovered [16]. Additionally:

- Postoperative rewarming strategies were developed
- Drugs against postoperative shivering were extensively tested
- Intraoperative warming devices were developed and evaluated
- Prewarming was described and evaluated.

Altogether this led to the publication of several national guidelines, e.g.:

- The National Institute for Health and Care Excellence (NICE) guideline [17]
- The American Society of Perianesthesia Nurses (ASPAN) guideline [18]
- The evidence-based guideline for prevention of perioperative hypothermia of the Canadian Association of General Surgeons [19]
- The German and Austrian guideline [20].

Introduction

Physiology of heat and cold sensation

To understand the core and peripheral temperature changes occurring during anaesthesia and surgery, a basic knowledge of the physiology of heat and cold sensation, thermo-regulation and heat exchange of the body is necessary. In this chapter, a brief and simplified overview of the physiology of heat and cold sensation is given. The following two chapters will give overviews of thermoregulation and heat exchange between the body and the environment.

> The physiology of heat and cold sensation, thermoregulation and heat exchange of the body are very complex. For the anaesthesia provider, not every detail is of clinical importance. A basic knowledge of the processes is sufficient.

Thermosensation is one the most ancient sensory processes and is present in all organisms [21]. In humans, the thermal information is generated by special thermo-receptors and transported to the brain using specialised nerve fibres and pathways.

Heat and cold sensation has at least four physiological functions:

1. The afferent heat and cold signals help to identify objects and materials through touch [22]. For example, metals can be easily discriminated from plastic with the help of the thermal information because metals have a high heat capacity and therefore stay cold longer in the hand compared to plastic.
2. The afferent heat and cold signals help to perceive a 'feeling' from the body if it is warm or cold. This is part of the general sense of the physiological condition of the body, also called interoception [23].
3. The afferent heat and cold signals help to detect potentially noxious thermal stimuli that pose a threat to the integrity of the skin (e.g. burns). Information about noxious temperature is detected and transported by different special thermoreceptors and nerve fibres from information about innocuous temperature.
4. The afferent heat and cold signals are signals for autonomic thermoregulation. The core body temperature of humans is tightly regulated under normal circumstances. To allow thermal regulation, adequate temperature sensing of the core of the body and the body surface is necessary.

> Thermoregulation is only one function of the sensation of heat and cold.

The following structures are involved in the process of heat and cold sensation:

1. Thermoreceptors
2. Thermosensitive neurons and their afferent nerve fibres
3. Neuronal pathways in the spinal cord and the brain
4. Special nuclei in the thalamus and hypothalamus
5. Cortex of the brain.

Thermoreceptors

Temperature is sensed in the free nerve endings of thermosensitive neurons by specific receptor proteins of the transient receptor potential (TRP) family of ion channels.

The TRP channels consist of six transmembrane protein domains. The functional channel is relatively non-selectively permeable to cations, including sodium, calcium and magnesium. The structure of one receptor protein (TRPV1) is shown in Fig. 2.1.

The basis of thermosensation lies in the property of these channels to conduct ions in a highly temperature-dependent manner.

In general, every biochemical reaction, every enzyme and ion channel, is to some degree temperature dependent. However, the steepness of this temperature dependence is different in distinct enzymes and ion channels and can be expressed and quantified using the dimensionless Q_{10} value. Q_{10} is defined as the relative change in reaction rate upon a 10 °C increase in temperature. Ion channels typically have a Q_{10} value between

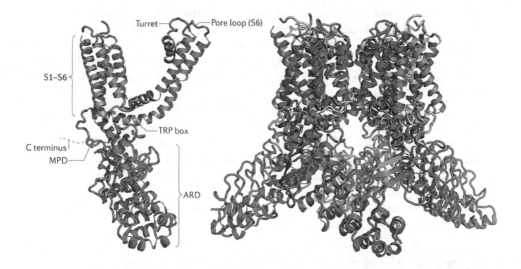

Nature Reviews | Neuroscience

Fig. 2.1 The structure of a transient receptor potential (TRP) V1. (Reprinted by permission from Macmillan Publishers Ltd: Vriens J, Nilius B, Voets T. Peripheral thermosensation in mammals. Nat Rev Neurosci 2014; **15**: 573–589 [21].)

2 and 3. This means, that a rise in temperature of 10 °C will increase the reaction rate by a factor of 2 or 3. Heat-activated ion channels exhibit a Q_{10} value of more then 7, whereas cold-activated channels display a Q_{10} value of less than 1, which means that the reaction rate drops during an increase in temperature [21].

Six of these TRP channels have been linked to temperature sensing ranging from noxious cold to noxious heat [24]. These thermoreceptors have the characteristic attribute that temperature alone can activate them; some by heat, others by cold. Every receptor type has a specific range of activating temperatures. However, some receptors can also be activated by molecules like capsaicin or menthol (Fig. 2.2).

Anktm1

Anktm1 is also called TRPA1 and plays a role as a chemical, mechanical and osmotic nociceptor and is also activated by temperatures below 17 °C. It is a prime candidate for transducing noxious cold signals [22].

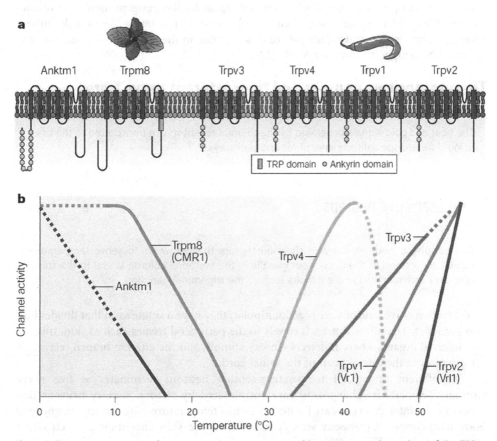

Fig. 2.2 Temperatures ranging from noxious heat to noxious cold activate several members of the TRP family. Some of the thresholds of activation and maximal activation are based on averaged values from different studies. Dashed lines indicate an uncertainty in the exact slope of the lines. (Reprinted by permission from Macmillan Publishers Ltd: Patapoutian A, Peier AM, Story GM, Viswanath V. ThermoTRP channels and beyond: mechanisms of temperature sensation. Nat Rev Neurosci 2003; **4**: 529–539 [24].)

Trpm8

The transient receptor potential melastatin receptor 8 (Trpm8 or TRPM8) is activated by temperatures below 26 °C and seems to be the most important receptor for sensing non-noxious cold, expressed in many thermosensitive neurons. It is also activated by agents known to produce the sensation of cold e.g. menthol and eucalyptol.

Trpv3 and Trpv4

Trpv (or TRPV) channels are also called vanilloid receptors. Trpv3 and Trpv4 are both activated by non-noxious warmth. The receptors have slightly different activation characteristics. Trpv3 is activated by temperatures above 33 °C and Trpv4 is activated by temperatures above 24 °C [22].

Trpv1 and Trpv2

Trpv1 and Trpv2 ion channels are involved in the transduction of noxious heat. Trpv1 is activated by temperatures above 43 °C and by capsaicin, the pungent ingredient of chili peppers [22]. The receptor is sensitised by inflammatory mediators like bradykinin and prostaglandin, demonstrating the role of this receptor in thermal hyperalgesia. Trpv2 is activated by temperatures above 52 °C [22].

Thermosensitive neurons and their afferent nerve fibres

The heat and cold signals generated by the thermal receptors are transported to the brain using different specialised nerve fibres and pathways.

Thermosensitive neurons

The peripheral neurons carrying thermoreceptors that allow us to sense temperature stimuli are located in the dorsal root ganglia in the vertebral column lateral to the spinal cord and within cranial nerve ganglia such as the trigeminal ganglion.

Thermosensitive neurons are pseudounipolar: they have a single axon that divides into two branches. The afferent branch travels to the peripheral tissues such as skin, mucosa and internal organs, where it detects sensory stimuli, and the efferent branch relays this information to the dorsal horn of the spinal cord.

The afferent branch of temperature-sensing neurons terminates as free nerve endings. Temperature changes that are encountered by visceral sensory neurons that innervate the internal organs are limited to a small temperature range around the normal body temperature. Cutaneous sensory neurons in the skin encounter a much larger temperature range (Fig. 2.3)[21, 24].

In the free nerve endings, the thermal information is coded in the form of action potentials.

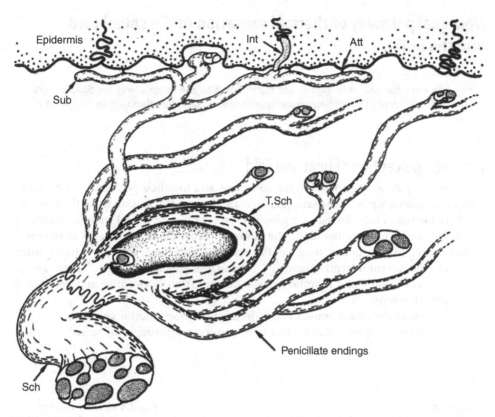

Fig. 2.3 Free nerve endings terminating in the skin. Sch = Schwann sheath of a preterminal nerve fiber carrying several unmyelinated axons. T. Sch. = terminal Schwann cell which gives origin to pencillate endings. The endings terminate either in the subepidermal corium (Sub) or intraepidermally (Int). Att = attachment between the basal laminae of the epidermis and the nerve ending. (Reproduced from: Cauna N. The free penicillate nerve endings of the human hairy skin. J Anat 1973; **115**: 277–288 [25] with kind permission by John Wiley & Sons Limited.)

In general, every thermosensitive neuron expresses only one type of thermoreceptor [24]. Thermosensitive neurons sensing cold signals have predominantly thinly myelinated Aδ-fibres with a conductive velocity of 9–15 m s^{-1}. In contrast, thermosensitive neurons sensing heat have predominantly unmyelinated C-fibres with a conductive velocity of 1 m s^{-1} [22]. Noxious cold- and heat-sensing neurons have thinly myelinated Aδ-fibres or C-fibres like other nociceptive neurons.

At comfortable skin temperatures cutaneous thermosensitive neurons fire action potentials continuously. Cooling of the skin increases cold receptor firing, whereas warming reduces the firing frequency of cold receptors until it ceases. In contrast, warming of the skin increases the firing frequency of warm receptors and decreases the firing frequency of cold receptors. Like mechanosensors of the skin, cold and warm receptors show pronounced adaptation when temperature is held constant after a sudden change. In contrast, thermosensitive neurons sensing noxious cold and heat are silent at thermoneutral temperature, but show a linear firing intensity as a reaction to noxious cold or heat and show little adaptation [21].

Neuronal pathway of thermal sensation in the spinal cord and the brain

The afferent heat and cold signals are transported to the brain using specialised nerve fibres and pathways. Depending on the specific physiologic function various pathways are utilised.

Localised perception of heat and cold

The simplest pathway is related to the conscious and localised perception of heat and cold information, e.g. when we are touching an object. Information from the thermo-sensitive neurons of the dorsal root ganglia is relayed via the dorsal root entry zone to the spinal cord and there mainly to the lamina I. The lamina I is located at the most dorsal aspect of the dorsal horn of the spinal cord. Here the nerve fibres form synapses with thermoreceptive lamina I cells in the spinal cord [21]. These lamina I cells are functionally and morphologically distinct from nociceptive and polymodal nociceptive neurons [26].

The axons of the spinal lamina I cells decussate via the anterior commissure to the contralateral lateral spinothalamic tract and then ascend through the spinal cord and

Fusiform NS
28–1007

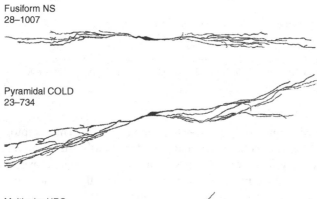

Pyramidal COLD
23–734

Multipolar HPC
24–514

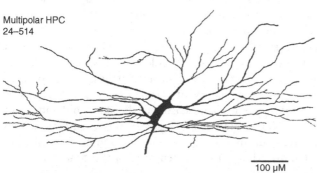

100 µM

Fig. 2.4 Reconstructions of nociceptive (NS), thermoreceptive (COLD) and polymodal nociceptive (HPC) sensory laminar I neurons. (Reprinted by permission from Macmillan Publishers Ltd: Han ZS, Zhang ET, Craig AD. Nociceptive and thermoreceptive lamina I neurons are anatomically distinct. Nat Neurosci 1998; **1**: 218–225 [26].)

the brainstem via the spinal lemniscus to a dedicated thalamocortical relay nucleus in the posterolateral thalamus – the posterior part of the ventromedial nucleus (VMpo) [27,28]. The axons of the trigeminal lamina I cells decussate in the brain stem to the contralateral side of the trigeminothalamic tract and ascend via the trigeminal lemniscus to another dedicated thalamocortical relay nucleus in the posterolateral thalamus – the posterior part of the ventromedial nucleus (VMb) [28].

From the posterolateral thalamus the filtered and processed information is relayed via the thalamocortical radiations to the primary sensory cortex, the gyrus postcentralis [27]. Here the conscious perception of temperature originates [21]. However, this pathway is only responsible for cutaneous thermal perception and is unlikely to contribute to thermal regulation and homeostasis.

The information from the thermosensitive neurons of the dorsal root ganglia is relayed via the contralateral lateral spinothalamic tract to the thalamus and then to the primary sensory cortex.

General sense of warm and cold

The pathway for the general sense of warm and cold is more complicated. It involves some of the already-mentioned structures and pathways, but additional structures are involved. Information from the thermosensitive neurons of the dorsal root ganglia and the trigeminal nerve is relayed via the thermoreceptive lamina I cells, the contralateral lateral spinothalamic tract and the trigeminothalamic tract to the posterolateral nuclei in the thalamus. From these nuclei, neurons project not only into the primary sensory cortex, but also into the dorsal posterior insular cortex.

The insula is a part of the brain hidden by the temporal lobe folded deep within the lateral sulcus separating the temporal lobe from the parietal and frontal lobes. It is involved in consciousness and plays a role in functions linked to emotion and homeostasis. The dorsal insular cortex contains a sensory representation, not only from temperature, but also from pain, itch, muscular and visceral sensations, sensual touch and other sensations from the body. This region seems to constitute a primary interoceptive image of homeostatic afferents [27]. From the dorsal posterior insula the temperature information is relayed to the mid-insula and then predominantly to the right anterior insula. The insula has very intimate connections with the anterior cingulate cortex, the amygdala and the hypothalamus [23]. The anterior cingulate cortex regulates the interaction between cognition and motor control in relation to changes in emotional and motivational states. Together with the amygdala it belongs to the limbic system, which is a complex set of brain structures that supports a variety of functions, including emotion, behaviour and motivation. This is thought to be the basis for the emotional assessment of temperature. This emotional assessment then causes affective motivational and behavioural thermoregulatory responses like moving into the shade, changing clothes and so on.

Furthermore, thermosensory information is transmitted from the spinothalamic tract and the trigeminal nerve to the lateral parabrachial nucleus in the brain stem, which is the main integration site for all homeostatic afferent activity, essential for the maintenance of cardiovascular, respiratory energy and fluid balances [23]. From the lateral parabrachial nucleus, information is relayed to the posterolateral nucleus VMb in the thalamus and to another thalamic nucleus, the ventral caudal portion of the medial dorsal nucleus. From that nucleus the thermal information is relayed directly to the anterior cingulate cortex [23]. The direct activation of the insula and the anterior cingulate cortex corresponds with the generation of both sensation, and motivation and drive behaviour [23].

> The general sense of warm and cold is relayed via the contralateral lateral spinothalamic tract to the thalamus and from the thalamus to the dorsal posterior insular cortex and the anterior cingulate cortex, the amygdala and the hypothalamus.

Perception of noxious heat and cold

Activation of sensory neurons relaying information of noxious heat and cold can activate motor neurons via spinal interneurons leading to a rapid withdrawal in response [21]. These neurons also form a dense network with autonomic cell columns in the spinal cord, thus forming a spino-spinal loop for somato-autonomic reflexes [23]. Additionally they are using the above-mentioned pathways to the primary sensory cortex, the insula and the limbic system.

> Noxious heat and cold signals can activate motor neurons leading to a rapid withdrawal in response.

Afferent signals for autonomic thermoregulation

As described above, the thermosensory information transmitted via the contralateral lateral spinothalamic tract and from the trigeminal nerve is relayed to the lateral parabrachial nucleus in the brain stem. From the lateral parabrachial nucleus information is also relayed to the anterior hypothalamus [23], especially to the preoptic nucleus [21] via the medial forebrain bundle [29]. The anterior hypothalamus also receives input from the spinohypothalamic tract that approaches the lateral anterior hypothalamus through the periventricular stratum [29].

The anterior hypothalamus itself also contains temperature-sensitive neurons, which not only respond to synaptic input from peripheral neurons, but also respond to small temperature changes in the brain [21]. Here the involuntary autonomic thermoregulatory processes like sweating, vasodilation, vasoconstriction and shivering are initiated.

> Thermosensory information is relayed to the anterior hypothalamus via the contralateral lateral spinothalamic tract and the lateral parabrachial nucleus in the brain stem. Here the involuntary autonomic thermoregulatory processes like sweating, vasodilation, vasoconstriction and shivering are initiated.

Chapter

3

Physiology of thermoregulation

The human thermoregulatory system relies primarily on behavioural thermoregulation and secondarily on autonomic responses for the maintenance of thermal homeostasis. This is because autonomic thermoregulation has only a limited capacity in preventing hyperthermia or hypothermia in extreme environments, whereas behavioural thermoregulation is a very powerful mechanism [30].

All thermoregulatory actions are controlled by several brain mechanisms in an organised manner to optimise the internal thermal environment of the core of the body for appropriate molecular activities and reactions by proteins, such as enzymes, receptors and ion channels.

Definition of the thermal core of the body

The thermal core of the body can be defined as those inner tissues whose temperatures are not changed in their relationship to each other by circulatory adjustments and changes in heat dissipation to the environment that affect the thermal periphery of the body [31].

In normal humans, the core temperature is preserved very well between 36.5 and 37.5 °C despite changing environmental conditions [32]. Core temperature varies depending on the circadian rhythm (Fig. 3.1). The lowest core temperatures are found during the night time and the highest in the early afternoon.

Behavioural or voluntary thermoregulation

Although it is well known that behavioural thermoregulation is very powerful [30], little is known about its neuroanatomy [34]. Many brain regions are involved in behavioural thermoregulation, like the insular, anterior cingulate, primary and secondary somatosensory and orbitofrontal cortex, and the amygdala, as well as the dorsomedial hypothalamus [30]. In general, behavioural thermoregulation depends more on peripheral thermal sensation than on central temperature [34]. This reflects the fact that behavioural thermoregulatory actions are often aiming at escaping the forthcoming thermal stress [34] or an anticipated thermal insult [30]. It is mainly driven by thermal comfort or discomfort [30].

Behavioural thermoregulation triggers conscious decisions in order to preserve the thermal balance whenever possible. Typical behavioural thermoregulatory responses alter the heat exchange of the body with the environment. These responses include behaviour

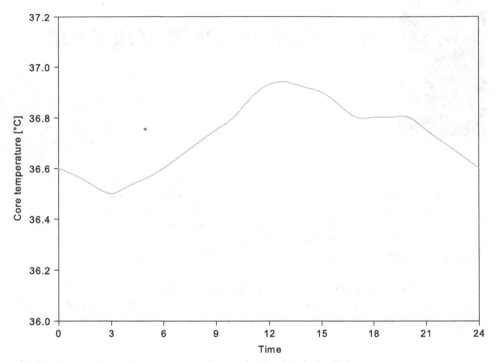

Fig. 3.1 The core temperature varies depending on the circadian rhythm [33].

such as searching for sunny, dry, warm and wind-sheltered environments and the avoidance of hostile thermal environments. Other options are the creation and application of different clothing or simply changing the temperature of the air conditioner or heating. Behavioural thermoregulation includes the conscious or unconscious decision to lower work rate or to end work to prevent the body from thermal injury or reaching a point of near collapse [30]. Behavioural thermoregulation also includes planning adequate insulation and suitable work under the expected thermal conditions, meaning that the person does not have to be already exposed to this environment.

Autonomic thermoregulation

Autonomic thermoregulatory responses are usually activated when the deep body temperature starts to change because behavioural thermoregulation was inadequate or could not be used sufficiently because of conflicting behavioural demands [30]. Therefore central thermosensors are more important for autonomic thermoregulation [34] than peripheral thermoreceptors. The most important regulatory centre of the autonomic thermoregulatory system is the hypothalamus. It can be divided into an anterior region, a middle region, a posterior region and a lateral region. For autonomic thermoregulation the anterior region with the preoptic nucleus is the most important.

The preoptic nucleus in the hypothalamus is the most important regulatory centre of the autonomic thermoregulatory system. This receives thermal information about core body and skin temperatures, and, in turn, induces involuntary autonomic thermoregulatory processes like sweating, vasodilation, vasoconstriction and shivering.

The preoptic nucleus in the anterior hypothalamus itself also contains temperature-sensitive and temperature-insensitive neurons. About 30% of the neurons of the preoptic nucleus of the anterior hypothalamus can be classified as warm-sensitive neurons [29] and only a few can be classified as cold sensitive. These warm-sensitive neurons are of utmost importance for thermoregulation and increase their firing rate with increasing temperature (Fig. 3.2) [29].

These neurons have a dendrite orientation that is ideal for the collection of incoming thermal information from the brainstem (Fig. 3.3) [34]. The medial dendrites are oriented perpendicularly, pointing to the periventricular region where they can receive information from the spinohypothalamic tract, which approaches the lateral anterior hypothalamus through the periventricular stratum [35]. The medial dendrites of the warm-sensitive neurons can reach the third ventricle and may receive chemosensitive information regarding endogenous substances in the cerebrospinal fluid of the third ventricle.

The lateral dendrites of the warm-sensitive neurons point to the medial forebrain bundle, which is another pathway for relaying thermal information to the anterior hypothalamus [35]. In this way preoptic warm-sensitive neurons act as integrators of thermal information. They are sensitive to their own temperature and also receive afferent information from the skin and other thermoreceptors within the body [34].

The fact that most of the temperature sensitive neurons are warm-sensitive is probably caused by the high brain temperature, which is much closer to the upper survival limit then to the lower limit [34]. Therefore, core overheating is much more dangerous than cooling [34] and must lead to an immediate and intense response. However, cold-sensitive neurons that

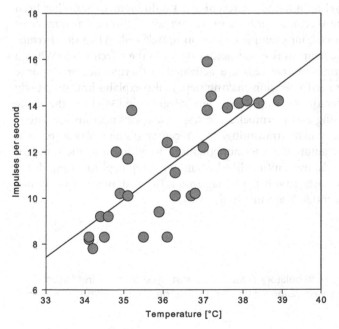

Fig. 3.2 Temperature-dependent firing rate of a warm-sensitive neuron in the anterior hypothalamus. Measured values and regression line [29].

Temperature Insensitive Neurones   **Warm Sensitive Neurones**

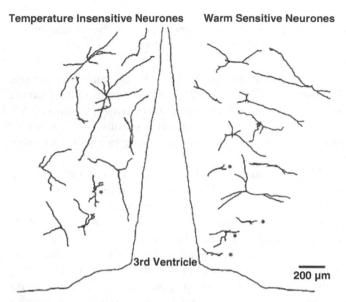

3rd Ventricle

200 µm

Fig. 3.3 Dendrite orientation of warm-sensitive neurons and temperature insensitive neurons in the anterior hypothalamus. (Reproduced from: Griffin JD, Saper CB, Boulant JA. Synaptic and morphological characteristics of temperature-sensitive and -insensitive rat hypothalamic neurones. J Physiol 2001; **537**: 521–535 [29] with kind permission by John Wiley & Sons Limited.)

increase their activity with a decrease of temperature have also been described. The cold sensitivity of these neurons seems to be due to excitatory and inhibitory synaptic input from nearby warm-sensitive neurons [34]. Their role is relatively unclear, because both heat-defence and cold-defence responses are initiated by changes in the activity of warm-sensitive neurons.

For a long time it was assumed that the information from the thermosensitive neurons is integrated via a network consisting of several neurons into some kind of mean body temperature. This temperature was then thought to be compared with an external or internal reference signal, generating a thermoeffector response [34]. However, this network has not yet been found. In recent years a different scenario has been proposed. In this model the thermosensitive neurons are wired through a number of other neurons to an effector cell, for example a skeleton muscle cell. When the thermosensitive cell is activated, the neurons fire and send a signal to the effector cell. When a large number of these thermosensitive cells are activated, a thermoeffector response occurs. This model does not need a decision-making step. It also explains how deep body temperatures and skin temperatures contribute to thermoregulation [34]. Over the whole process of temperature sensing and thermoeffector response many neurons and interneurons are involved. Thereby many transmitter and receptor systems play a role and can influence the process of autonomic thermoregulation. In addition to the transient receptor potential ion channels, transmitters like histamine, norepinephrine [36], dopamine, 5-hydroxytryptamine, acetylcholine, prostaglandin E_1, and neuropeptides like orexin A and B, and neuropeptide Y are involved.

Effector responses

The principal autonomic thermoregulatory defences against hyperthermia and hypothermia in humans include skin vasomotor activity, non-shivering thermogenesis, shivering and sweating [37].

Heat loss is normally regulated without the major responses of sweating or shivering because cutaneous vasodilation and vasoconstriction are usually effective enough. A second reason that sweating or shivering are activated last is that these effectors are either water-consuming or energy-consuming [34] and these resources are normally well protected. Efferent pathways to thermoeffectors have not been well characterised in humans yet. Each effector has its own pathway and needs a unique combination of signals from peripheral and central thermoreceptors [34].

In the following paragraphs, thermoregulatory vasoconstriction, shivering and non-shivering thermogenesis will be discussed. Thermoregulatory vasodilatation and sweating will not be covered because they are not of interest in the context of perioperative hypothermia.

Autonomic cold-defence responses

Autonomic cold responses are triggered by massive thermal exposures that lead to a decrease in deep body temperature [30]. Even very small decreases in core temperatures of about 0.1 °C are enough to trigger autonomic thermoregulatory vasoconstriction. This core temperature is very often termed the threshold for thermoregulatory vasoconstriction. If core temperature decreases more than 1 °C, thermoregulatory shivering is induced. However, peripheral skin temperatures also contribute to the threshold of thermoregulatory vasoconstriction and shivering. The influence of skin temperature is estimated to be about 20%.

Vasoconstriction
Purpose of thermoregulatory vasoconstriction

Thermoregulatory vasoconstriction decreases cutaneous heat loss and constrains metabolic heat to the core of the body.

Therefore, skin perfusion has not only a nutritional component but also a thermoregulatory component [32]. Thermoregulatory vasoconstriction changes skin perfusion mainly in acral regions, e.g. fingers, toes and nose, where arteriovenous shunts are located [32]. Without thermoregulatory vasoconstriction these shunts are fully dilated and blood flow is much higher than the metabolic demand of this region. The high blood flow is used to dissipate metabolic heat from the body to the environment. However, at typical ambient temperatures in the operating room, shunt flow is reduced to a minimum [32]. The arteriovenous shunts are constricted via α_1-receptors by norepinephrine released from sympathetic nerves [38]. The decreasing skin perfusion reduces the skin temperature and thereby limits the temperature gradient between the skin and the environment and reduces heat loss (Fig. 3.4).

As a second mechanism of thermoregulatory vasoconstriction, venous return of the blood from the arms and the legs is directed from the superficial veins to the deep veins. Here the venous blood exchanges heat with the arterial blood on a counter-current principle. This mechanism helps maintain the temperature of the core of the body, whereas the heat content of the arms and the legs decreases.

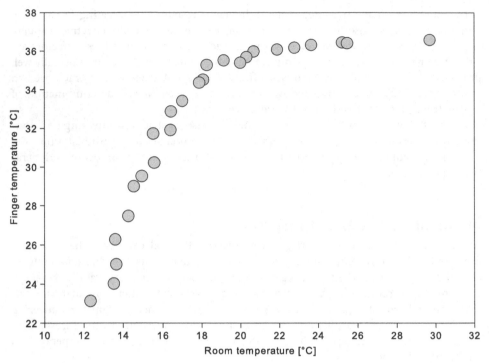

Fig. 3.4 Skin temperature at the index finger depending on the room temperature. In this volunteer experiment, lowering of the room temperature induced thermoregulatory vasoconstriction. It can clearly be seen that the lower room temperatures lead to a decrease in the skin temperature of the fingertip, thereby limiting the temperature gradient between the room and the finger.

Measurement of thermoregulatory vasoconstriction

Thermoregulatory vasoconstriction can be measured with venous-occlusion volume plethysmography at the finger [39], laser Doppler technology [40] or a forearm–fingertip temperature gradient [40]. The last method is the simplest technically and is applied in most clinical studies. With this method thermoregulatory vasoconstriction is measured by calculating the skin surface temperature gradient of the forearm minus the fingertip temperature. The forearm temperature is measured at the radial side of the arm midway between the wrist and the elbow and the fingertip temperature is measured on the tip of the index or middle finger opposite the nail bed [40]. Without thermoregulatory vasoconstriction the skin temperature at the finger is slightly higher than the forearm skin temperature, because there is no insulating fat tissue at the fingertip. This means that the forearm fingertip gradient is negative. When the gradient increases above 0 °C, thermoregulatory vasoconstriction has begun. At a gradient of more than 4 °C significant vasoconstriction is present.

Neuronal pathway of thermoregulatory vasoconstriction

If thermoregulatory vasoconstriction is triggered, the warm–sensitive neurons from the anterior hypothalamus activate different neuron groups in the midbrain via the medial forebrain bundle [34]. The information is then relayed to cells from the raphe/pyramidal

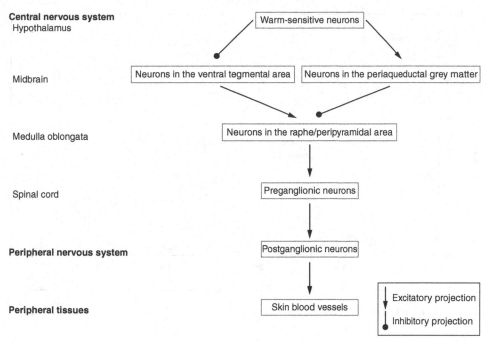

Fig. 3.5 Schematic drawing of the neuronal pathway of thermoregulatory vasoconstriction. (Drawing modified after [34].)

area of the medulla and these neurons activate the sympathetic preganglionic neurons in the intermediolateral column [34]. After the postganglionic neurons have been activated, arteriovenous shunts constrict (Fig. 3.5).

Shivering
Purpose of thermoregulatory shivering

Normal thermoregulatory shivering is a last-resort defence that is activated only when behavioural compensations and maximal arteriovenous shunt vasoconstriction are insufficient to maintain core temperature. Thermoregulatory shivering is an involuntary, oscillatory muscular activity that augments metabolic heat production.

Vigorous shivering can increase metabolic heat production by up to 600% above basal level [37]. However, thermoregulatory shivering is not a very effective method of remaining warm or of rewarming, because shivering also increases heat loss.

Measurement of thermoregulatory shivering

Thermoregulatory shivering can be graded using several different clinical scales:
- Grade 0: No tremor activity
- Grade 1: Intermittent activity
- Grade 2: Vigorous, continuous activity [41].

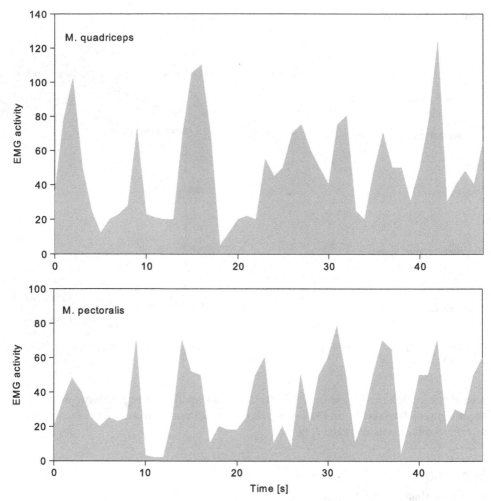

Fig. 3.6 Shivering activity in electromyography (EMG). The slow waxing-and-waning pattern in the different muscles can be seen. (Redrawn and modified from [43].)

Another scale from Guffin [42] uses four grades:

- Grade 0: No shivering
- Grade 1: Occasional mild tremors in the jaw and neck
- Grade 2: Intensive tremors in the chest
- Grade 3: Continuous violent muscle activity

The scales show that thermoregulatory shivering starts with an intermittent activity usually at the head, neck and chest.

Shivering activity can also be identified and quantified using electromyography. The fundamental tremor frequency on the electromyogram in humans is typically near 200 Hz.

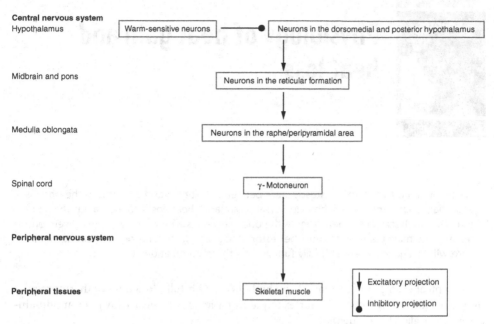

Fig. 3.7 Schematic drawing of the neuronal pathway of thermoregulatory shivering. (Drawing modified after [34].)

This basal frequency is modulated by a slow, 4–8 cycles min^{-1}, waxing-and-waning pattern (Fig. 3.6).

Neuronal pathway of thermoregulatory shivering

The efferent pathway for shivering involves disinhibition of tonically inhibited neurons [34]. Normally the preoptic nucleus of the anterior hypothalamus sends inhibitory signals via the medial forebrain bundle to the posterior hypothalamus to inhibit shivering. The pathway then runs from the posterior hypothalamus through the midbrain and the pons, and activates cell groups in the reticular formation [34]. Cells from the raphe/pyramidal area of the medulla directly and indirectly activate the γ-motorneurons and α-motorneurons of the ventral horn of the spinal cord [34]. Spinal motorneurons and their axons are the final path for shivering (Fig. 3.7).

Non-shivering thermogenesis

Non-shivering thermogenesis can increase the heat production of newborns that have relatively large deposits of brown adipose tissue. It is probably essential for the survival of human newborns under normal conditions [44]. Under control of the hypothalamus, norepinephrine is released from the sympathetic nerves in the brown adipose tissue and induces a cascade of events leading to lipolysis of triacylglycerols and thus to a release of free fatty acids [44]. The free fatty acids are then combusted in the mitochondria, which are endowed with tissue-specific uncoupling protein-1 that permits combustion unhindered by oxidative phosphorylation [44]. This leads to a large thermogenic response. However, in adults [37] and infants [37,45], non-shivering thermogenesis does not play a role during anaesthesia.

Physiology of heat gain and heat loss

To maintain normothermia, a steady state between heat gain and heat loss in the body is essential. Short imbalances between heat gain and heat loss do not alter the core temperature because the periphery of the body serves as a thermal buffer. However, long term, a thermal steady state must be restored. Otherwise cooling or overheating of the core will take place, even with fully functioning thermoregulation.

A typical example of cooling of the body even with fully functioning thermoregulation is accidental hypothermia, for example in patients with near drowning, mountaineering or avalanche accidents.

Passive overheating occurs in persons exposed to massive heat and is called hyperthermia, for example malignant hyperthermia. In contrast to hyperthermia, fever is not a passive phenomenon. Fever is caused by a regulated increase in core temperature and involves the coordination of a wide range of autonomic, endocrine and behavioural responses.

Heat gain

The body can gain heat from heat production within the body or from external sources.

Heat production within the body

Heat production within the body is generated as a by-product of all metabolic processes. In a resting person, the heat production is equal to the energy expenditure and can be measured by indirect calorimetry. Energy expenditure is linked to oxygen consumption and carbon dioxide production, and can be calculated according to the formula by Weir [46]:

$$EE = \left(3.9\,\dot{V}O_2 + 1.1\,\dot{V}CO_2\right) 1.44 \left[\min \text{kcal}\,d^{-1}\,ml^{-1}\right] \qquad (4.1)$$

where

EE = energy expenditure [kcal d^{-1}]
$\dot{V}O_2$ = oxygen consumption [ml min^{-1}]
$\dot{V}CO_2$ = carbon dioxide production [ml min^{-1}]

Energy expenditure should nowadays be expressed in watts ($1\text{ W} = 1\text{ J s}^{-1}$). To convert the results to watts [W] the value must be divided by 20.62.

The energy expenditure of an individual varies throughout the day. During the morning hours the energy expenditure rises, whereas during the night-time it is lower. The following factors increase energy expenditure:

- Male sex
- Young age
- Postovulatory phase of the menstrual cycle
- Nutrition intake
- Cold climate
- Attention and emotions
- Smoking
- Pregnancy and lactation
- Hyperthyreosis.

The following factors decrease energy expenditure:

- Female sex
- Older age
- Fasting
- Sleep
- Hypothyreosis.

The basal energy expenditure (in the morning hours, resting and fasting) can be estimated by the formula of Harris and Benedikt (1919) (Fig. 4.1) [47].

Basal energy expenditure of men is:

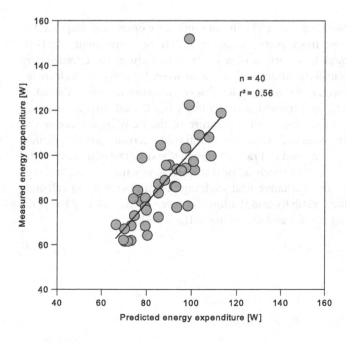

Fig. 4.1 Predicted and measured basal energy expenditure of 40 adult patients. There is an acceptable correlation between the predicted and the measured values. However, in the individual, large deviations are possible.

$$BMR = 66.473 + 13.7516W + 5.0033H - 6.755A \tag{4.2}$$

Basal energy expenditure of woman is:

$$BMR = 655.0955 + 9.5634W + 1.8496H - 4.6756A \tag{4.3}$$

where
BMR = basal metabolic rate in kcal day^{-1}
W = weight in kg
H = height in cm
A = age in years

Examples:

A 45-year-old man, 185 cm tall and weighing 90 kg has an estimated basal energy expenditure of 1926 kcal d^{-1} = 93 W.

A 84-year-old woman, 163 cm tall and weighing 53 kg has an estimated basal energy expenditure of 1071 kcal d^{-1} = 52 W.

In a perioperative patient without anaesthesia, heat production in the body can be estimated to be roughly 1 W kg^{-1}.

Heat gain from external sources

In addition to heat production within the body, heat can also be gained from external heat sources. Heat can be transfered by radiation, convection or conduction.

Heat gain by radiation

Heat can be gained from a radiative source like the sun or a large operating lamp. Heat is transferred by emission of electromagnetic radiation at infrared wavelengths (0.1–10 μm) from the radiating object to a surface of a lower temperature. Heat transfer by radiation requires no heat transfer medium such as air or water [48]. When electromagnetic radiation strikes an object, radiation is either absorbed, transmitted or reflected. If it is reflected or transmitted no heat transfer occurs. Only when the infrared electromagnetic radiation is absorbed it can raise the temperature of the body by increasing the energy of the molecules of the object. The fraction of infrared electromagnetic radiation that is absorbed is called emissivity and can range between 0 and 1. The emissivity of the human skin is 0.98, which means that nearly all heat transferred by infrared electromagnetic radiation is absorbed [48]. Radiative heat exchange is cumbersome to calculate because it is a function of the emissivity and the fourth power of the absolute temperature in kelvin of the radiating surface and absorbing surface [48]:

$$\dot{Q}_R = \varepsilon\sigma \left(K_1{}^4 - K_2{}^4 \right) A \tag{4.4}$$

where
$\dot{Q}_R$ = radiative heat exchange [W]
ε = emissivity
σ = Stefan Boltzmann constant = 5.67 10^{-8} W m^{-2} K^{-4}

K_1 = surface temperature of the radiating surface [K]
K_2 = surface temperature of the radiated surface [K]
A = heat exchanging area [m^2]

In the perioperative period, heat gain by radiation does not play a relevant role, except when a radiating lamp or radiating ceiling is used as an active warming therapy [49–51].

Heat gain by convection

Heat can be gained from a convective heat source like a forced-air warmer. Heat is transferred by convection directly from molecule to molecule, thereby increasing the molecular energy of the warmed surface and thus the temperature. Convective heat exchange is associated with molecular displacement. The displaced molecules diffuse along their energy (temperature) gradient from high to low temperatures [48]. When molecular displacement is due only to the temperature gradient, the process is called natural or free convection. When molecular displacement is also due to an external force (e.g. increased air velocity when using a hair dryer) it is called forced convection [48]. Therefore, convective air warmers are also called forced-air warmers.

Convective heat transfer can be described as follows:

$$\dot{Q}_C = h_c \Delta T\, A \tag{4.5}$$

where
$\dot{Q}_C$ = convective heat exchange [W]
h_C = heat exchange coefficient for convection [W $m^{-2}\,°C^{-1}$]
ΔT = temperature gradient between the warming medium and the surface [°C]
A = heat exchanging area [m^2]

In the perioperative period, heat gain by convection plays a role when a forced-air warmer is used.

Heat gain by conduction

Heat can be gained from a conductive heat source like a water mattress under the back. Heat is transferred by conduction from molecule to molecule, which increases molecular energy and, therefore, temperature, but does not cause molecular displacement like heat transfer by convection. Conduction occurs only in or between solids, because the strong intermolecular bonds prevent molecular displacement. Conductive heat transfer can be described as follows [48]:

$$\dot{Q}_K = h_K \Delta T\, A \tag{4.6}$$

where
$\dot{Q}_K$ = conductive heat exchange [W]
h_K = heat exchange coefficient for conduction [W $m^{-2}\,°C^{-1}$]
ΔT = temperature gradient between the warmer and colder surface [°C]
A = heat exchanging area [m^2]

In the perioperative period, heat gain by conduction plays a role when a conductive warming mattress is used [52].

Heat loss from the body

To be in a thermal steady state, the body must lose all the heat that is generated by the metabolism and added by external sources, otherwise the body would overheat. Heat is lost from the body surface by radiation, convection, conduction and evaporation. Heat is also lost via the airways by evaporation and convection.

Heat loss by radiation and convection

Heat loss from the body occurs mainly from surfaces that are exposed to the surrounding air. For practical reasons, the heat exchange via radiation and convection can be calculated together (Fig. 4.2). Heat transfer can be described as follows [48, 53]:

$$\dot{Q}_{RC} = h_{RC} \, \Delta T \, A \tag{4.7}$$

where
$\dot{Q}_{RC}$ = convective and radiative heat exchange [W]
h_{RC} = heat exchange coefficient for radiation and convection [W m^{-2} °C^{-1}]
ΔT = temperature gradient between the room and the body surface [°C]
A = heat exchanging area [m^2]

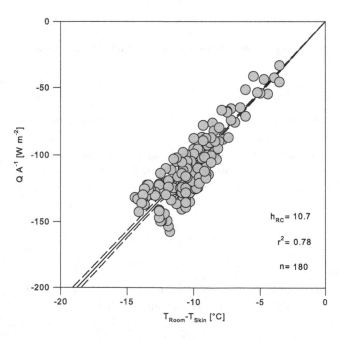

Fig. 4.2 Determination of the combined heat exchange coefficient for radiation and convection of a volunteer. Measured values and regression line with confidence intervals. (Reproduced from: Bräuer A, English MJM, Sander H, Timmermann A, Braun U and Weyland W. Construction and evaluation of a manikin for perioperative heat exchange. *Acta Anaesthesiol Scand* 2002; **46**: 43–50 [53] with kind permission of John Wiley and Sons Inc.)

h_{RC} = 10.7

r^2 = 0.78

n = 180

Under perioperative conditions these heat losses are most important, because the heat exchanging area is very large.

Heat loss by conduction

Heat loss from the body by conduction occurs only in areas were the body has direct contact to a solid body like the ground or an operating table. In clinical practice, heat loss by conduction is very small, because the areas involved are small and the thermal conductivities are low [48]. Conductive heat loss can be calculated as described above.

Under perioperative conditions, these heat losses are only of minimal importance, because the heat exchanging area is very small. The conductive heat losses from the back to an operating table can be estimated to be about 3 to 5 W [54].

Heat loss by evaporation from the skin

Heat loss by evaporation occurs because heat is needed to provide the energy for a change of state from liquid to vapour. The vapour molecules then diffuse along the energy gradient from high to low vapour pressure. The heat exchange of evaporation is a function of the vapour pressure gradient and the air velocity, analogous to convection. The driving gradient for the evaporation of water from the skin is the partial pressure of water vapour between the skin and the surrounding air. Heat loss by evaporation can be calculated as follows [48]:

$$\dot{Q}_E = h_E \, \Delta p \, A \tag{4.8}$$

where
$\dot{Q}_E$ = evaporative heat loss [W]
h_E = heat exchange coefficient for evaporation [W m^{-2} kPa^{-1}]
Δp = partial pressure gradient of water vapour between the skin and the surrounding air [kPa]
A = heat exchanging area [m^2]

Heat losses by evaporation from the skin can be divided into sensible evaporation, which means visible sweating, and insensible evaporation. Under perioperative conditions, sweating normally does not play a role. The physiological heat losses by insensible evaporation from the skin are also not of great importance and can be estimated to be roughly 10% of the radiative and convective heat losses. Although this may be an invalid estimation, it is used very often in clinical studies, because insensible evaporation from the skin cannot be measured by simple techniques [55].

In the perioperative setting, evaporative heat losses from the skin are not of great importance and can be estimated to be about 10% of the radiative and convective heat losses.

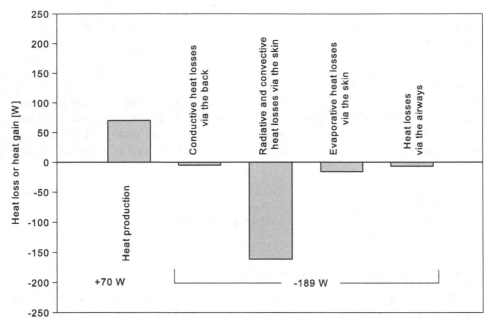

Fig. 4.3 Calculated heat balance for a minimally dressed person under the typical conditions of an operating room.

Heat losses from the airways

Heat losses from the airways can be divided into convective heat losses and evaporative heat losses. In general, these heat losses are of minor importance compared to heat losses by convection and radiation from the skin. Model calculations and measurements from patients show consistently that heat losses from the airways are about 7–10 W [56], with the convective heat loss being about 1 W and the evaporative heat loss about 6 W [56].

Heat losses from the airways are of minor importance.

Heat balance

Calculating the heat gain and heat loss for a minimally dressed person under the conditions of an operating room with a room temperature of about 22 °C gives the heat balance shown in Fig. 4.3.

It can be clearly seen that the heat loss outweighs the heat gain from body heat production. This means that a normal person exposed to this environment can only maintain normothermia by activating autonomic thermoregulatory vasoconstriction.

Influence of body weight on the heat balance

Obese persons have a problem losing heat because their high body mass leads to a high energy production roughly proportional to their weight. Because weight increases faster than surface area as body size increases, larger patients lose a smaller fraction of their heat production [57]. In contrast, slim persons have a problem maintaining their body heat content, because their heat production is lower and the body surface area is relatively large.

Chapter

5

Influence of preanaesthetic core temperature and premedication

Development of perioperative hypothermia starts before patients enter the operating room.

Preanaesthetic core temperature

A low preanaesthetic core temperature is a risk factor for the development of intraoperative and postoperative hypothermia [58–60]. There are only a few large studies giving the core temperature of patients before induction of anaesthesia. In the study by Mitchell and Kennedy [61], the median core temperature before induction of anaesthesia was 36.4 °C. Many patients had only a core temperature of 36.1 or 36.2 °C (Fig. 5.1).

Interestingly, the incidence of hypothermia before induction of anaesthesia was about 1%, although the patients were not premedicated. In the study by Mehta and Barclay [60], about 5% of all patients were already hypothermic before they left the ward and Frank *et al.* [62] found the incidence was in the same range.

The patient's core temperature should be measured and documented before the patient goes to the operating room [16, 63] or on admission to the operating room [17].

Risk factors for a low preanaesthetic core temperature

Age

Under normal conditions younger and older patients have comparable core temperatures (Fig. 5.2).

However, older patients show an attenuated thermoregulatory vasoconstriction under cold stress [65] and surveys of body temperatures in elderly people living at home found deep body temperatures below 35.5 °C in 10% of those studied. Elderly patients also show delayed thermoregulatory vasoconstriction under anaesthesia [66]. Low core temperatures of older patients can sometimes be observed before induction of anaesthesia and are probably caused by pre-existing chronic diseases (e.g. diabetes mellitus with diabetic neuropathy [67]) and chronic medication.

Extreme low weight

Malnourished patients with anorexia nervosa have a considerable risk of being hypothermic [68,69]. In a study by Jonas *et al.* [68], 10 of 23 patients were hypothermic with a core

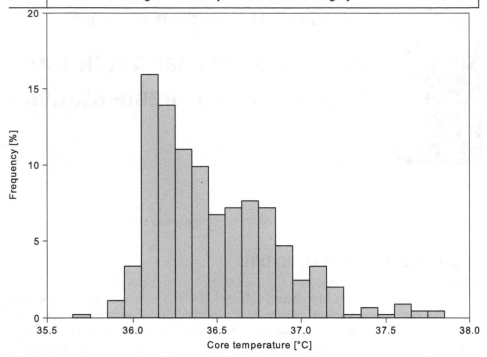

Fig. 5.1 Core temperature of 446 patients before induction of anaesthesia. (Redrawn after [61].)

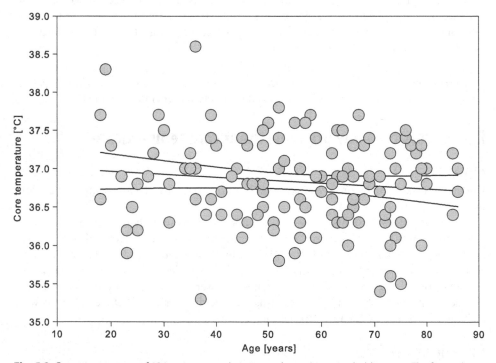

Fig. 5.2 Core temperatures of 126 patients on admission to the preoperative holding area. The figure shows the measured values and regression line with confidence intervals. There is only a minimal decrease in mean core temperature with age. (Reproduced from Bräuer A, Waeschle RM, Heise D, *et al.* Preoperative prewarming as a routine measure. First experiences. *Anaesthesist* 2010; **59**: 842–850 [64] with permission of Springer.)

temperature below 36 °C, whereas in another study the mean core temperature of anorectic patients was 35.2 °C [69].

Other pre-existing diseases

There are several rare diseases that are associated with an increased risk of impaired thermoregulation. In patients with one of these diseases, preanaesthetic core temperature can be below 36 °C. These diseases include:

- Severe hypothyreosis
- Diabetes mellitus with diabetic neuropathy [67]
- Tetraplegia and paraplegia
- Hypothalamic injury or tumour
- Shapiro syndrome
- Infantile neuronal lipofuscinosis
- Periodic spontaneous hypothermia
- Thymoma
- Poikilothermia syndrome and some other rare diseases.

Influence of chronic medication

Chronic medication can influence preanaesthetic core temperature and intraoperative temperatures. This has been shown for chronic medication with antidepressants [70]

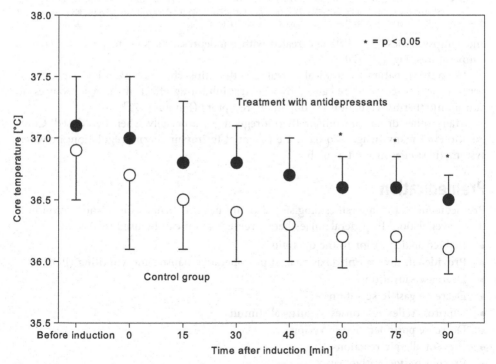

Fig. 5.3 Perioperative core temperatures of patients chronically treated with antidepressants vs. a control group. The figure shows the mean values and standard deviation. (Redrawn after [70].)

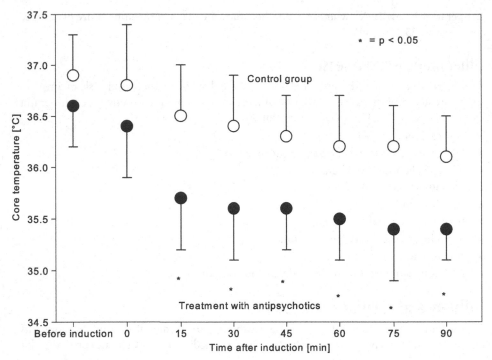

Fig. 5.4 Perioperative core temperatures of patients chronically treated with antipsychotics vs. a control group. The figure shows the mean values and standard deviation. The patients treated with antipsychotics have a lower core temperature compared to the control group. (Redrawn after [71].)

and antipsychotics [71]. Patients treated with antidepressants tend to have higher core temperatures (Fig. 5.3) [70].

In contrast, patients chronically treated with antipsychotics have a lower core temperature which seems to be caused by a central inhibiting effect of these substances on autonomic thermoregulation via dopamine receptors (Fig. 5.4) [71].

Many other drugs can impair thermoregulation, especially when overdosed. Combinations of many drugs also have the potential to impair thermoregulation; however, systematic studies are not available.

Premedication

Premedication by anaesthesiologists also influences behavioural and autonomic thermoregulation. In general, anaesthetic premedication can be used to:

- Reduce anxiety prior to the operation
- Provide effective prophylaxis against postoperative nausea and vomiting (PONV)
- Decrease salivation
- Decrease gastric secretions
- Suppress reflex responses to surgical stimuli
- Decrease postoperative shivering
- Prevent allergic reactions
- Prevent postoperative pain
- Decrease anesthetic requirements for the surgical procedures.

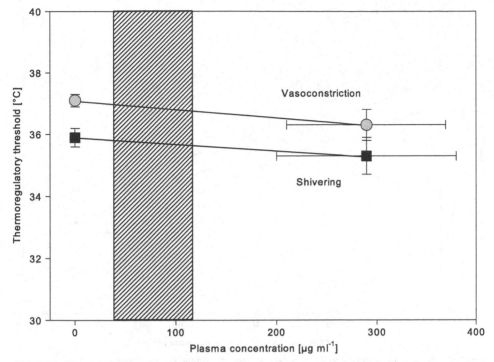

Fig. 5.5 Influence of midazolam on thermoregulatory vasoconstriction threshold and thermoregulatory shivering threshold. The thresholds decrease slightly with increasing plasma concentrations of midazolam. The figure shows the mean values and standard deviation. The hatched area symbolises the range of plasma concentrations of midazolam in adult premedicated patients. (Redrawn and modified from [39].)

However, anaesthetic premedication is handled very different in daily practice. The most popular goals for premedication are to reduce anxiety, to provide prophylaxis against PONV and to decrease salivation. Many patients are premedicated with benzodiazepines, whereas other patients do not receive premedication at all.

Drugs to reduce anxiety or to cause tranquillity
Benzodiazepines
Benzodiazepines and especially midazolam are very often prescribed to reduce anxiety prior to surgery and are effective. It can be assumed that this anxiolytic and sedative treatment influences behaviour and thereby attenuates behavioural thermoregulation. The influence of midazolam on autonomic thermoregulation has been studied by Kurz *et al.* [39]. In this study they tested the influence of a plasma concentration of about 300 ng ml^{-1} of midazolam. This is much more than the plasma concentrations that are reached in adult patients premedicated with 10 mg of midazolam p.o., who usually show plasma concentrations of below 150 ng ml^{-1}. They found that midazolam does not produce substantial inhibition of autonomic thermoregulation. The threshold for thermoregulatory vasoconstriction decreased only about 0.3 °C, suggesting that patients premedicated with midazolam will maintain nearly normal core temperatures in typical hospital environments until induction of anaesthesia (Fig. 5.5) [39].

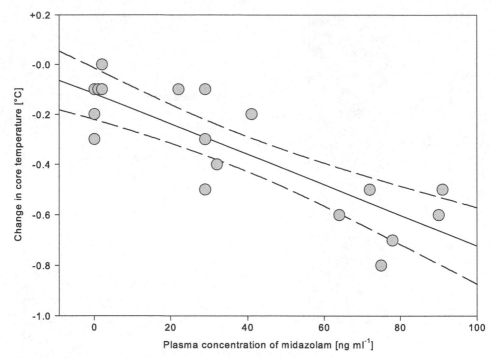

Fig. 5.6 Influence of midazolam on the core temperature of volunteers. With increasing plasma concentrations of midazolam the decrease of core temperature is getting larger. The figure shows the measured values and regression line with confidence intervals. (Redrawn and modified from [72].)

In contrast to these data, other studies show an influence of premedication on the preoperative core temperature. In a volunteer study by Matsukawa *et al.* [72], premedication with midazolam caused a dose-dependent decrease in core temperature of up to 0.8 °C, which was probably caused by an initial redistribution of heat from the core of the body to the periphery, because the volunteers were vasoconstricted before premedication and vasodilated after premedication. The effect on core temperature was pronounced when the volunteers were more sedated (Fig. 5.6).

This is also true for other benzodiazepines, e.g. flunitrazepam (Fig. 5.7).

The effect of benzodiazepines to drop the core temperature can be attenuated by forced-air warming, high room temperatures or atropine.

> Premedication with benzodiazepines can lead to a clinically relevant drop in core temperature before induction of anaesthesia.

Clonidine

Clonidine is also given commonly for premedication because it produces sedation and analgesia, decreases sympathetic activity, blunts the haemodynamic response to intubation, and reduces anaesthetic requirements during surgery. The influence of different doses of clonidine given orally on autonomic thermoregulation has been studied in

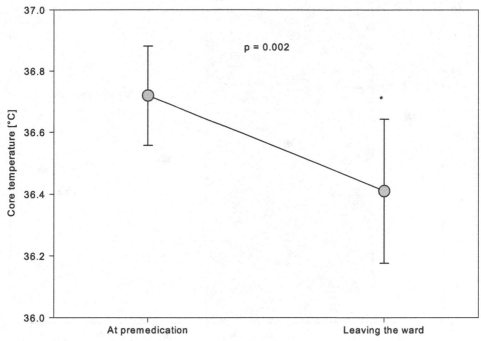

Fig. 5.7 Influence of 1 mg flunitrazepam on the core temperature of ten cardiac surgical patients. A significant decrease in core temperature can be seen after premedication before patients have even left the ward. The figure shows the mean values and standard deviation.

volunteers [73]. Clonidine reduced the threshold for vasoconstriction and shivering in a dose-dependent way (Fig. 5.8). In general, the influence was comparable with that of midazolam.

However, in a clinical trial with a premedication of 150 μg of clonidine p.o., no influence on the preoperative core temperature was observed. In theory, clonidine should have a more pronounced effect on preoperative core temperature compared to midazolam. It is unclear why the clinical data show the opposite.

Drugs to reduce postoperative nausea and vomiting

Postoperative nausea and vomiting (PONV) is a common and distressing complication associated with anaesthesia surgery. Many studies have shown that prophylactic low-dose dexamethasone or 5-HT$_3$ receptor antagonists like ondansetron or dolasetron are effective. To date no data about the influence of low-dose dexamethasone on core temperatures are available. Ondansetron shows no influence on vasoconstriction and shivering thresholds in volunteers, although it is well known that 5-HT$_3$ receptor antagonists reduce postoperative shivering [74].

Premedication with drugs to reduce PONV does not lead to a clinically relevant drop in core temperature.

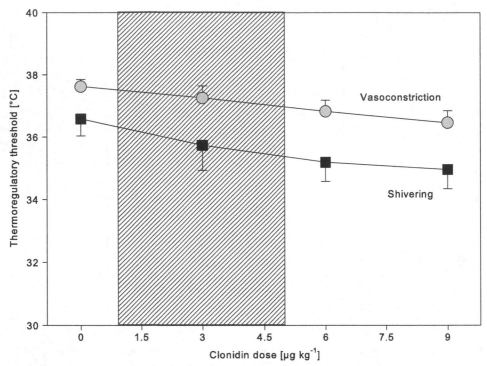

Fig. 5.8 Influence of clonidine on thermoregulatory vasoconstriction threshold and thermoregulatory shivering threshold. The thresholds decrease with increasing plasma concentrations of clonidine. The figure shows the mean values and standard deviation. The hatched area symbolises the range doses used for premedication in adult patients. (Drawn using data from [73].)

Anticholinergic drugs

Anticholinergic drugs can decrease salivation and reduce vagal reactions during induction of anaesthesia. The effect of benzodiazepines on drop of core temperature can be attenuated by co-administration of atropine [75].

Opioids

Opioids are sometimes used as a premedication to reduce preoperative pain and to help to reduce postoperative pain. Autonomic thermoregulation is attenuated by opioids and the vasoconstriction threshold is reduced [76–78] suggesting that patients premedicated with opioids will be at risk of having a lower core temperature at induction of anaesthesia.

> Premedication with opioids can lead to a clinically relevant drop in core temperature before induction of anaesthesia.

Histamine-receptor antagonists

Histamine-receptor antagonists were sometimes given as a premedication to reduce gastric juice secretion and to reduce the gastric juice volume and acidity. One study reported that premedication with the H_2 receptor antagonist famotidine augmented intraoperative hypothermia, whereas another study could not find an influence. However, the topic is no longer of interest because proton pump inhibitors have replaced histamine-receptor antagonists for that indication.

> In general, special care should be taken to keep patients comfortably warm when they are given premedication (for example midazolam or opioids) [16] because premedication has the potential to reduce core temperature and to augment perioperative hypothermia.

Chapter

6

Influence of transportation to the operating room and preparation for surgery

In addition to premedication [71], the surgical environment is the next thermal stressor for the patient.

On the normal ward it is normally no problem for patients to maintain their body temperature (Fig. 6.1). The wards are comfortably warm and insulation, e.g. clothing or a hospital duvet, can be added according to the individual need of the patient. Before leaving the normal ward, patients have to remove their clothes and change into a hospital gown. The hospital gown together with a normal blanket is not sufficient to maintain a

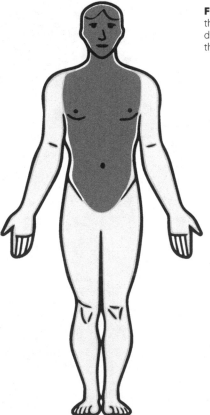

Fig. 6.1 Cartoon showing the temperature distribution in the body under normal conditions. Body temperature is not distributed evenly. The core of the body is warmer than the periphery of the body. (Figure created by Thomas Schulze.)

thermal steady state because the insulating properties of these materials are not good enough. The heat loss of the patient can be considerable during transfer to the operating room through long and cold hospital corridors.

Therefore the body loses a significant amount of heat and thermoregulatory vasoconstriction is activated. The core of the body maintains its temperature, but the heat content of the arms and legs decreases [79–81]. This means that an important temperature gradient between the core of the body and the periphery is created.

It is important to understand that a temperature gradient between the core and the periphery is nothing pathological. Under normal conditions there is always a temperature gradient between the core and the periphery of the body. This gradient is necessary to maintain thermal steady state conditions for the body, because the body must lose all the heat that is generated by the metabolism or it would overheat. To enable heat transfer from the core of the body to the environment, heat has to flow from the core to the periphery and then to the environment. A heat flow from the core to the periphery of the body is only possible when a temperature gradient exists between these compartments, because heat always flows from a site of higher temperature to a site of lower temperature. This temperature gradient changes over time and even a large temperature gradient is not pathological because the periphery of the body serves as a thermal buffer. Under cold stress the gradient is larger, whereas under heat stress it is smaller.

However, before induction of anaesthesia, this temperature gradient is of great clinical importance, because a large temperature gradient will cause a large redistribution of heat from the core of the body to the periphery after induction of anaesthesia or neuraxial anaesthesia [80–82]. This is a very important mechanism for the development of perioperative hypothermia.

Chapter

7

Influence of general anaesthesia

> Anaesthesia is the main risk factor for the development of perioperative hypothermia. It is much more important than the surgical procedure.

The induction of anaesthesia causes a drop in core temperature by:
- The influence of the anaesthetic drugs on thermoregulation
- Redistribution of heat from the core of the body to the periphery
- Vasodilatation
- Reduction of heat production.

Thermoregulation is also influenced by the positioning of the patient and positive pressure ventilation with positive end expiratory pressure (PEEP).

Influence of the anaesthetic drugs on autonomic thermoregulation

The human thermoregulatory system relies primarily on behavioural thermoregulation and only secondarily on autonomic responses for the maintenance of thermal homeostasis. Therefore, it is clear that every anaesthetic drug will impair thermoregulation. General anaesthesia removes the patient´s ability to regulate body temperature through behaviour, so that the less powerful autonomic defences alone are available to respond to changes in temperature [83]. However, autonomic thermoregulation is also impaired by anaesthetic drugs in a significant way.

In volunteer and clinical studies, the influence of anaesthetic drugs on autonomic thermoregulation was quantified by the shift in thresholds for thermoregulatory sweating, vasoconstriction and shivering. Sweating is irrelevant in the context of hypothermia and will not be discussed.

A thermoregulatory threshold can be defined as the core temperature at which this thermoregulatory response is triggered. This approach has the advantage that it gives a single number to describe the threshold. However, both core and skin temperatures contribute to the control of thermoregulatory responses. Therefore this threshold is ideally calculated to a designated mean skin temperature to be more precise [84]. Another problem is that volunteer and clinical studies of patients might give different results because surgical stimulation may facilitate thermoregulatory responses [85]. In an early trial by Washington *et al.* [85], the influence of painful electrical stimulation on thermoregulatory thresholds was tested. In this crossover trial the threshold for vasoconstriction

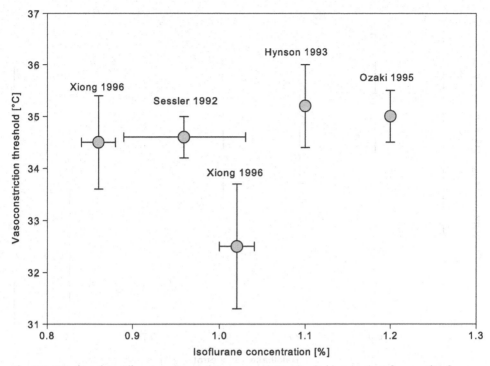

Fig. 7.1 Data from four different studies on the vasoconstriction threshold under the influence of isoflurane. Due to the different methods and situations used, the effect of isoflurane on thermoregulatory vasoconstriction is blurred. The figure shows the mean values and standard deviation. (Drawn using data from [86–88].)

was measured in five anaesthetised volunteers by using a forearm–fingertip temperature gradient of more than 4 °C as a parameter for significant vasoconstriction. They found that painful electrical stimulation slightly increased the threshold for significant vasoconstriction, but the difference was not statistically significant, with a p value of 0.050. It can be assumed that a more painful stimulation or a sixth volunteer could have resulted in significant differences. All this makes the comparison of the results of different studies cumbersome and can give the wrong impression (Fig. 7.1).

But what is the relevant threshold? Is it the vasoconstriction threshold determined in an extremely well-controlled volunteer trial? Or the vasoconstriction threshold determined in surgical patients during the operation? If the main interest is the effect of the anaesthetic drug on autonomic thermoregulation without other interferences, the threshold determined in volunteer trials gives the best answer. If the main interest is the clinical impact of the anaesthetic drug, the clinical data from patients under anaesthesia and surgery are probably more relevant. Therefore, in the following sections volunteer data and clinical data of patients under anaesthesia and surgery are reported separately.

Volatile anaesthetics

Volatile anaesthetics can be a significant factor for the development of perioperative hypothermia. The main reason for this is the attenuation of autonomic thermoregulation in the hypothalamus [36] and the spinal cord by volatile anaesthetics. In isolated perfused rat brain slices, halothane, for example, reduces the firing rate and thermosensitivity of

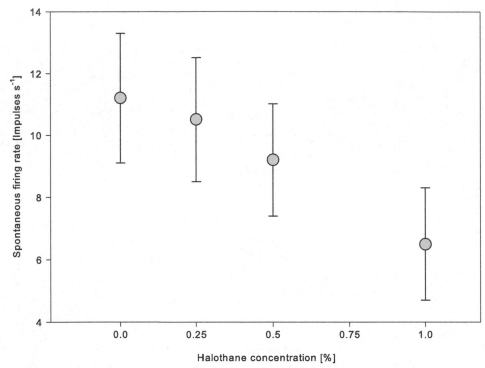

Fig. 7.2 Spontaneous firing rate of warm-sensitive neurons in the preoptic area of the hypothalamus of a rat brain slice with halothane concentration. The figure shows the mean values and standard error of the mean. (Drawn using data from [89].)

warm-sensitive neurons in the preoptic area of the hypothalamus in a dose-dependent way (Fig. 7.2) [89].

Volatile anaesthetics also increase the local release of norepinephrine in the preoptic area of the hypothalamus, which is associated with hypothermia during anaesthesia [36].

Halothane

Halothane is nowadays mainly of historical interest and no controlled volunteer studies are available on the influence of halothane on vasoconstriction and shivering threshold. In clinical studies, a concentration of 1% halothane (1.5 MAC) reduced the vasoconstriction threshold to 36.5 °C under orthopaedic surgery [90] or to 34.4 °C in patients undergoing donor nephrectomy [40]. In children undergoing urologic surgery 0.8% (1 MAC) reduced the vasoconstriction threshold to 35.5 °C and in children undergoing hypospadia repair 0.9% halothane (1.1 MAC) reduced the vasoconstriction threshold to 35.7 °C [91].

Enflurane

Enflurane is probably also more of historical interest. However, one volunteer study on the effect of enflurane on vasoconstriction threshold is available. In the study by Washington *et al.* [85] 1.3% enflurane (0.75 MAC) reduced the threshold for significant thermoregulatory vasoconstriction to 35.1 °C. In a subsequent patient study during

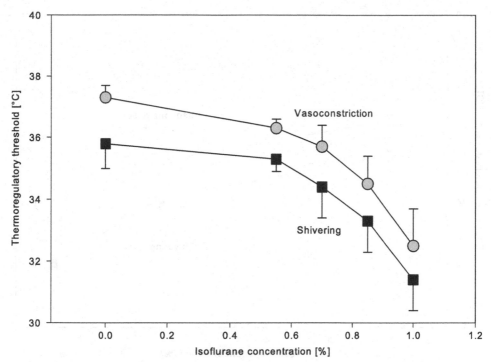

Fig. 7.3 Influence of increasing doses of isoflurane on the thermoregulatory thresholds of vasoconstriction and shivering. The figure shows the mean values and standard deviation (Drawn using data from [86].)

colorectal surgery, 0.8% enflurane (0.5 MAC) reduced the threshold for significant thermoregulatory vasoconstriction to 35.6 °C [92].

Isoflurane

The influence of isoflurane on thermoregulation has been studied very well in volunteers [86, 92] and patients [66, 87]. Probably the most informative study on the effect of isoflurane on the thresholds for thermoregulatory vasoconstriction and shivering is that by Xiong *et al.* [86]. In this study it is clearly shown that isoflurane has a dose-dependent effect on the thermoregulatory thresholds and that this effect is not linear. With high concentrations of isoflurane the thresholds decreased disproportionally more (Fig. 7.3).

With 1% isoflurane (0.8 MAC) the vasoconstriction threshold decreased to 32.5 °C. Higher concentrations were not studied in this trial, although they are used in clinical practice. It must be assumed that the thresholds would further decrease with higher concentrations of isoflurane.

In clinical studies of patients undergoing surgery, the vasoconstriction threshold with 1.2% isoflurane (1 MAC) was only reduced to 35.0–35.1 °C [66, 87], which is significantly higher than 32.5 °C. This is probably due to two main reasons:

1. The enhancement of autonomic thermal responses by surgical stimulation [86].
2. No correction for the effects of skin temperature on thermoregulation [86].

However, patients anaesthetised with higher concentrations of isoflurane (1.8 MAC) have a significantly greater decrease in core temperature than patients anaesthetised

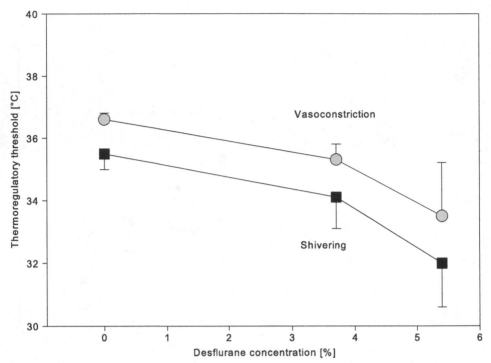

Fig. 7.4 Influence of increasing doses of desflurane on the thermoregulatory thresholds of vasoconstriction and shivering. The figure shows the mean values and standard deviation. (Drawn using data from [94].)

with lower concentrations of isoflurane (1 MAC) [93]. This indicates that in surgical patients a dose-dependent effect of isoflurane on the thermoregulatory thresholds exists that is relevant. The combination of isoflurane and nitrous oxide leads to a higher threshold for vasoconstriction [87].

Desflurane

The influence of desflurane on thermoregulation has been studied in volunteers [94] and patients. The most informative study on the effect of desflurane on the thresholds for thermoregulatory vasoconstriction and shivering is the study by Annadata *et al.* [94]. This study shows clearly that desflurane also has a dose-dependent effect on the thermoregulatory thresholds and that this effect is not linear. With high concentrations of desflurane the thresholds decreased disproportionally more (Fig. 7.4). This is the same effect as described for isoflurane.

In a clinical study with patients undergoing ENT surgery, the vasoconstriction threshold with 6% desflurane was 35 °C, which is once again significantly higher than the vasoconstriction threshold in volunteers. The reasons for this are probably the same as for isoflurane.

Sevoflurane

Although sevoflurane is one of the frequently used modern volatile anaesthetics, its influence on thermoregulation has not been studied in volunteers. However, some clinical data are available indicating that in surgical patients 1 MAC of sevoflurane has the same effect on the vasoconstriction threshold as 1 MAC of isoflurane, with a vasoconstriction threshold of 35.1 °C [87]. The combination of 0.5 MAC sevoflurane and 0.5 MAC nitrous oxide leads to a higher threshold for vasoconstriction of 35.8 °C.

All the volatile anaesthetics studied have a non-linear dose-dependent effect on the thermoregulatory thresholds. With high concentrations of volatile anaesthetics the thresholds decrease disproportionally more.

In clinical studies with patients undergoing surgery, the vasoconstriction thresholds are higher, due to the enhancement of autonomic thermal responses by surgical stimulation [86]. However, the thresholds are all below 36.0 °C so that thermoregulatory vasoconstriction under volatile anaesthesia cannot prevent perioperative hypothermia.

Propofol

In volunteers, propofol shows a dose-dependent effect on the thermoregulatory thresholds (Fig. 7.5) [84]. In contrast to volatile anaesthetics, propofol linearly reduces the vasoconstriction and shivering thresholds.

Clinical studies of patients undergoing surgery are not available, because propofol alone has no analgesic effect. The clinical studies of anaesthesia with propofol and opioids are presented in the paragraph about the influence of opioids on thermoregulation.

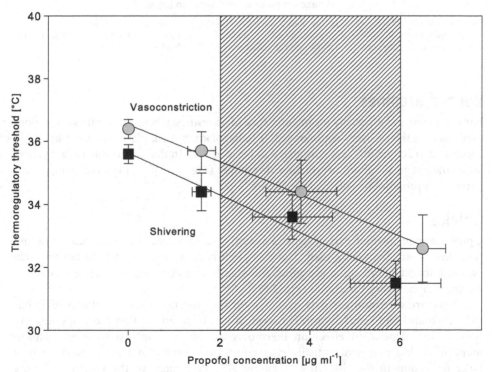

Fig. 7.5 Influence of increasing doses of propofol on the thermoregulatory thresholds of vasoconstriction and shivering. The figure shows the mean values and standard deviation. The hatched area shows the range of propofol plasma concentrations that are considered to be relevant. (Drawn using data from [84].)

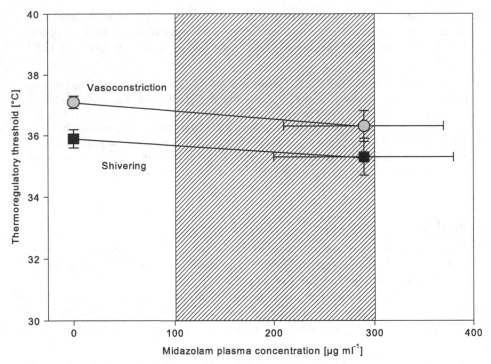

Fig. 7.6 Influence of midazolam on the thermoregulatory thresholds of vasoconstriction and shivering. The figure shows the mean values and standard deviation. The hatched area shows the range of midazolam plasma concentrations that are considered to be adequate. (Drawn using data from [39].)

Benzodiazepines

For induction and especially for maintenance of anaesthesia, benzodiazepines are seldom used because the recovery is prolonged. If midazolam is used, plasma concentrations of about 100 to 300 ng ml^{-1} are considered to be adequate. In this range, midazolam causes little changes in the thermoregulatory thresholds (Fig. 7.6) [39], especially when compared with propofol or volatile anaesthetics.

Opioids

Opioids are an integral part of general anaesthesia: fentanyl, alfentanil, sufentanil and remifentanil are frequently used. However, well-controlled volunteer studies are only available for alfentanil and meperidine. Alfentanil has a linear dose-dependent effect on the thermoregulatory thresholds (Fig. 7.7).

There are no volunteer data available on the thermoregulatory effects of fentanyl, sufentanil and remifentanil. However, it can be assumed that these opioids also have a dose-dependent effect on thermoregulation. In contrast to these opioids, meperidine has a special antishivering effect that results, at least in part, from a large reduction in the shivering threshold [77] compared to the reduction in the vasoconstriction threshold. This may result from κ–receptor activation at the level of the spinal cord by meperidine [77].

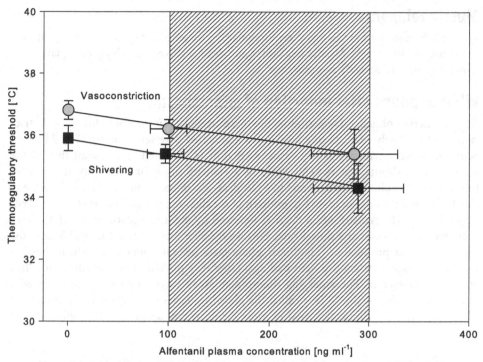

Fig. 7.7 Influence of alfentanil on the thermoregulatory thresholds of vasoconstriction and shivering. The figure shows the mean values and standard deviation. The hatched area shows the range of alfentanil plasma concentrations that are considered to be adequate. (Drawn using data from [76].)

In a clinical study of patients undergoing elective, donor nephrectomy with nitrous oxide/fentanyl anaesthesia, the vasoconstriction threshold was 34.2 °C [95]. In another clinical study in patients undergoing neurosurgical procedures, the vasoconstriction threshold with propofol/fentanyl anaesthesia was 34.5 °C. In children undergoing abdominal surgery, the vasoconstriction threshold with propofol/fentanyl anaesthesia was about 36 °C [45]. In patients undergoing surgery with total intravenous anaesthesia with propofol and remifentanil vasoconstriction thresholds of 35.0 [96] to 35.7 °C [96] were observed. Interestingly, the incidence of postoperative shivering is much higher in patients given total intravenous anaesthesia with remifentanil compared to e.g. alfentanil without any difference in core temperature. The higher incidence of postanaesthetic shivering is thought to reflect acute opioid tolerance and stimulation of N-methyl-D-aspartate (NMDA) receptors [97] and is not an effect of remifentanil on the shivering threshold.

All the intravenous anaesthetics studied have a dose-dependent effect on the thermoregulatory thresholds and, in contrast to volatile anaesthetics, this effect is linear. In clinical studies with patients undergoing surgery, the vasoconstriction thresholds are higher than in volunteer studies. However, the thresholds are all below 36.0 °C, so that thermoregulatory vasoconstriction under intravenous anaesthesia cannot prevent perioperative hypothermia.

Muscle relaxants

Muscle relaxants do not change thermoregulatory thresholds because they cannot pass the blood–brain barrier. Muscle relaxants can prevent shivering, which may play a role when patients are severely hypothermic.

What happens after induction of anaesthesia?

After induction of general anaesthesia, the thermoregulatory threshold for vasoconstriction is immediately reduced to a level below the actual core temperature (Fig. 7.8). The activated tonic thermoregulatory vasoconstriction is inhibited and vasodilation of the arteriovenous shunts occurs. This leads to a redistribution of heat from the core of the body to the colder periphery and to a fast decrease in core temperature. This phase in the development of perioperative hypothermia is called the *redistribution phase* and lasts about 1 hour. The redistribution phase is followed by the *linear phase*, in which the core temperature decreases at a slower rate. This decrease occurs because the body's heat loss exceeds its heat production. The linear phase lasts several hours, after which thermoregulatory vasoconstriction is activated again, because the core temperature is now low enough to trigger it. The emerging thermoregulatory vasoconstriction keeps the core temperature stable again. This is called the *plateau phase* of perioperative hypothermia [83]. These phases will be discussed in more detail in the following paragraphs.

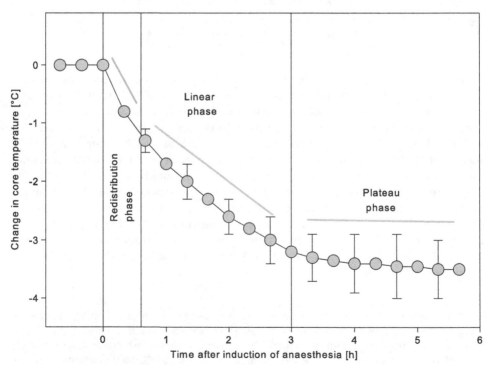

Fig. 7.8 Influence of induction of general anaesthesia on the core temperature. The redistribution, linear and plateau phases can be seen. The figure shows the mean values and standard deviation. (Redrawn with modifications from [98].)

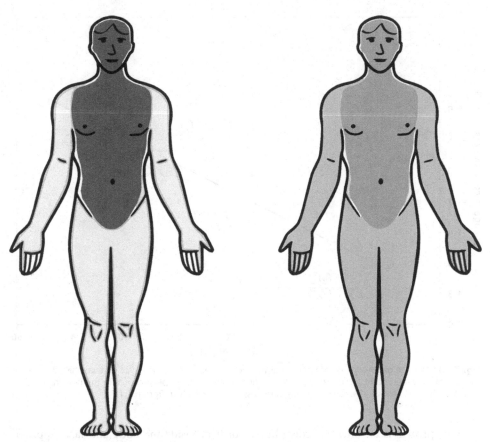

Fig. 7.9 Influence of induction of general anaesthesia on the distribution of heat inside the body. (Redrawn with modifications from [98] by Thomas Schulze.)

Redistribution phase

When patients arrive in the operating room in a hospital gown and covered with a normal blanket, they have already lost a significant amount of heat because the insulating properties of these materials are not high enough. Thermoregulatory vasoconstriction is activated and maintains the core temperature, but the heat content of the arms and legs is slowly decreasing, creating a large temperature gradient between the core of the body and the periphery [79, 80]. If patients are premedicated with a benzodiazepine their core temperature may already be reduced [72].

Induction of general anaesthesia reduces the thermoregulatory threshold for vasoconstriction below the actual core temperature. The activated tonic thermoregulatory vasoconstriction is now inhibited and vasodilation of the arteriovenous shunts occurs. Additionally, the more or less pronounced direct vasodilating effect of most anaesthetic drugs causes additional vasodilation, allowing the heat that was constrained to the thermal core of the body to flow down the temperature gradient into the colder peripheral tissues [98]. The temperature of the core decreases and the temperature of the peripheral tissues increases (Fig. 7.9).

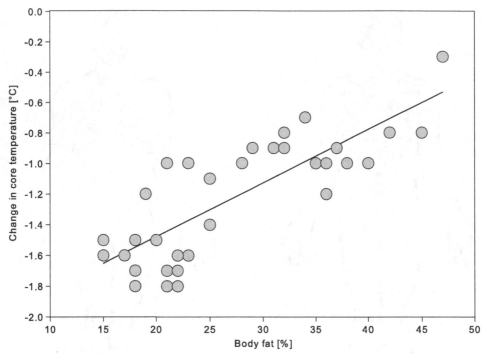

Fig. 7.10 Influence of body morphology on redistribution of heat after induction of general anaesthesia. The size of the drop in core temperature during the first hour is inversely proportional to the percentage of body fat. The figure shows measured values and regression line. (Redrawn from [57].)

This process is an internal redistribution of heat inside the body and lasts approximately 1 hour. The resulting change in core temperature from redistribution does not represent heat loss to the environment. Of course, parallel to this redistribution process, heat loss to the environment occurs, but during the redistribution phase the influence of environmental heat losses on core temperatures is of minor importance for the change in core temperature [80]. The magnitude of the change in core temperature due to redistribution of heat can vary considerably: in the volunteer study by Matsukawa *et al.* [80] it was 1.6 °C, whereas in clinical studies the drop in core temperature during the first hour of anaesthesia varies. Many studies have reported a drop in core temperature in this period of between 1.5 °C [99–101] and 0.1 °C [102, 103] or even not at all [104]. The factors influencing the magnitude of core temperature change due to redistribution are manifold.

The most important factor is the temperature of the peripheral tissues: the higher it is, the smaller the magnitude of redistribution will be, because this directly depends on the temperature gradient between the core and the periphery of the body. This temperature gradient is the driving force for the redistribution of heat. If – hypothetically – there was no temperature gradient there would be no redistribution of heat. The peripheral tissue temperature depends largely on the environmental conditions. After long exposure to a cold environment the peripheral tissues are cold [80], whereas after prewarming of the patient the peripheral tissues are warmer [79].

Another important factor is body morphology (Fig. 7.10) [57]. Obese patients have a high weight-to-body-surface ratio and thus generally have difficulty dissipating sufficient heat to the environment. This leads to vasodilation and a high peripheral tissue temperature, consequently reducing the magnitude of core temperature change after induction of anaesthesia [57].

In contrast to adults, newborns, babies and infants have a higher mass in the torso [98] and relatively little mass in their extremities. Therefore redistribution of heat contributes less to the drop in core temperature after induction of anaesthesia.

The magnitude is also influenced by haemodynamic changes. Vasodilation during induction of anaesthesia increases the drop in core temperature [99, 101] because vasodilation facilitates heat flow from the core of the body to the periphery. The use of vasoconstrictors like phenylephrine [101] or ephedrine during induction of anaesthesia reduces the magnitude of redistribution. A high cardiac output also increases the magnitude of redistribution of heat because it also enhances heat flow from the core of the body to the periphery. Consequently, the use of β-blockers can reduce the magnitude of redistribution.

A final factor can be warming therapy after induction of anaesthesia. Active warming therapy started immediately after induction of anaesthesia warms up the periphery, thus increasing the peripheral temperature. In adult patients this will not play a significant role, however in newborns and babies it can be effective enough to prevent any drop in core temperature after induction of anaesthesia [104].

> The magnitude of redistribution of heat increases with low temperature of the peripheral tissues (long exposure to cold, no prewarming), vasodilation during induction of anaesthesia and high cardiac output.
> The magnitude of redistribution of heat is reduced by a high temperature of the peripheral tissues (prewarming, obesity), minimal vasodilation during induction of anaesthesia and low cardiac output.

Linear phase

The linear phase follows the redistribution phase and lasts approximately 2 hours. During this phase, redistribution of heat inside the body is still going on, but is becoming less important. In the linear phase, heat losses exceeding the heat production of the body are getting more and more important (Fig. 7.11) [98]; heat production is reduced by 15–40% [98]. In contrast, heat losses by radiation, convection, conduction and evaporation increase, with heat losses by radiation and convection being the most important.

In obese patients, the cooling rate during the linear phase is slower probably due to the insulating capacity of adipose tissue [57]; it is higher in children and during large operations [98].

> In the linear phase, redistribution of heat becomes less important. The change in core temperature is mainly determined by heat losses exceeding heat production.

Plateau phase

The last phase of the typical intraoperative temperature curve is the plateau phase. It develops after the linear phase and can only be seen during longer operations after approximately 3 hours. The core temperature plateau can be passive or active. A passive core temperature plateau results from a new thermal steady state when heat

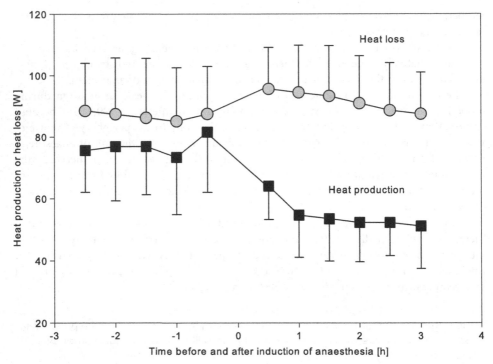

Fig. 7.11 Heat production and heat loss before and after induction of anaesthesia. After induction the heat losses increase slightly, whereas heat production is significantly decreased. The figure shows the mean values and standard deviation. (Recalculated and redrawn with data from [80].)

production equals heat loss without activating thermoregulatory defences. The fact that heat production is lowered by general anaesthesia, whereas heat losses are higher during anaesthesia and surgery means that such a passive plateau rarely develops without warming therapy [98]. During small operations with good insulation a passive temperature plateau can be reached [103]; during larger operations it can only be attained by active warming therapy, when heat production plus heat gain from the warming therapy equals the heat losses.

An active core temperature plateau develops after the core temperature has decreased sufficiently that thermoregulatory vasoconstriction is activated (Fig. 7.12). Once triggered, thermoregulatory vasoconstriction slows down the cooling rate dramatically. In some cases, core temperature does not decrease further or may even increase slowly. As a consequence, the core remains warmer than the periphery, thus restoring a new core-to-peripheral tissue temperature gradient. The heat content and tissue temperature of the arms and the legs still decreases [55]. This means that an active core temperature plateau does not represent a thermal steady state and that the mean body temperature decreases further.

In some patients no active core temperature plateau can be seen, because thermoregulatory vasoconstriction does not develop during anaesthesia [95]. Additionally, in patients receiving a massive transfusion without adequate warming of the blood, severe hypothermia can occur even when thermoregulatory vasoconstriction is activated. Another possibility for a drop in core temperature after an active core temperature plateau has been achieved is the deflation of a tourniquet. The release of a tourniquet is

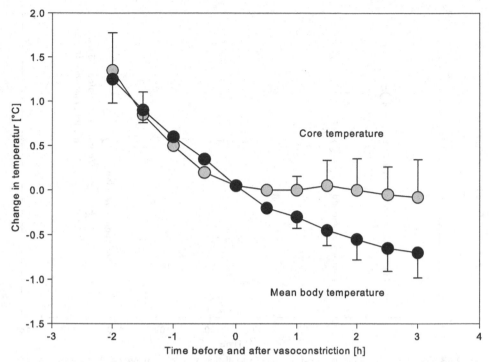

Fig. 7.12 Core and mean body temperatures before and after vasoconstriction. After vasoconstriction the core of the body maintains its temperature, whereas the mean body temperature still decreases due to the ongoing heat losses from the arms and the legs. The figure shows the mean values and standard deviation. (Redrawn using data from [55].)

associated with redistribution of heat from the core of the body to the cold, previously not perfused, extremity and a substantial core temperature drop can be observed (Fig. 7.13) [105].

Positioning of the patient and mechanical ventilation with positive end expiratory pressure (PEEP)

Thermoregulation serves as a switchboard of autonomic and endocrine control [106], and several non-thermal influences on thermoregulation can be observed. Therefore, positioning of patients in the operating room can influence vasoconstriction threshold and can modify the magnitude of perioperative hypothermia.

Positioning patients with their legs up can decrease the thermoregulatory threshold of vasoconstriction by more than 1 °C [107, 108]. This is thought to be an effect of baroreceptor loading of the heart by increasing the venous return and increasing the transmural pressure of the right atrium. As a consequence of this, thermoregulatory vasoconstriction is activated at a lower core temperature, leading to lower core temperatures at the end of the operation [108]. In contrast, an upright position leads to baroreceptor unloading and the vasoconstriction threshold is higher.

In other clinical studies it was shown that baroreceptor unloading by applying PEEP during mechanical ventilation increases thermoregulatory vasoconstriction threshold [96, 109].

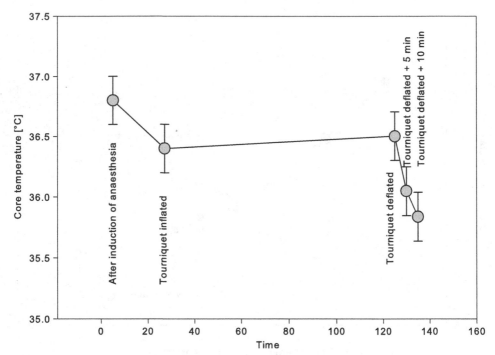

Fig. 7.13 Core temperature before and after tourniquet inflation and deflation. After deflation a second redistribution of heat can be seen in the drop in core temperature. The figure shows mean and standrd error. (Redrawn using data from [105].)

Concluding remarks

In this chapter, several influences on thermoregulation have been discussed. It is obvious that every general anaesthetic abolishes behavioural thermoregulation and general anaesthesia also impairs autonomic thermoregulation. Vasoconstriction and shivering thresholds are shifted to lower core temperatures. During anaesthesia and surgery, thermoregulatory thresholds are always below 36 °C. Therefore thermoregulatory vasoconstriction limits the magnitude of hypothermia, but cannot prevent perioperative hypothermia. What are the consequences of these data?

1. Patients undergoing surgery under general anaesthesia need active warming therapy to maintain normothermia.
2. As all anaesthetic drugs cause hypothermia, the choice of drugs should not rely on the influence of drugs on thermoregulation.
3. Redistribution of heat is very important in the initial phase of anaesthesia and should be reduced by prewarming of the patient; otherwise the patient can be hypothermic before surgery begins.
4. Anaesthetic depth should be adequate because too deep anaesthesia causes more hypothermia [93].
5. Tourniquet release causes a second redistribution of heat. This should be anticipated.

Chapter

8

Influence of regional anaesthesia

In this chapter, the influence of regional anaesthesia without the additional use of sedation on the development of perioperative hypothermia is discussed. This is often called the 'wide awake approach', in contrast to regional anaesthesia with sedation.

> Regional anaesthesia can also lead to perioperative hypothermia, especially neuraxial anaesthesia, which produces thermal perturbations that may be as large or even larger than those observed during general anaesthesia [98]. Core temperature should therefore also be measured during neuraxial anaesthesia.

Neuraxial anaesthesia

Pathophysiology

The induction of neuraxial anaesthesia causes a drop in core temperature by:

- Vasodilatation and redistribution of heat from the core of the body to the legs [98]
- The thermal imbalance between heat production and heat loss [110]
- The influence of the neuraxial anaesthesia on thermoregulation [98].

In contrast to general anaesthesia, heat production is not decreased by neuraxial anaesthesia. It can even rise as an attempt to maintain core temperature [110].

Spinal and epidural anaesthesia are commonly used anaesthetic techniques for many operative procedures. The pathophysiology of hypothermia development in both methods is very similar so that both methods will be described together. However, it seems that hypothermia occurs a few minutes faster with spinal anaesthesia compared to epidural anaesthesia due to the faster onset of spinal anaesthesia [111].

Redistribution of heat

After injection of the local anaesthetic into the subarachnoid or epidural space, the anaesthetic blocks the transmission of afferent nerve signals and efferent motor neurons. As a consequence, neuraxial anaesthesia inhibits the already activated tonic thermoregulatory vasoconstriction of the cold-exposed patient in the part of the body affected by the block. Vasodilation of the arteriovenous shunts occurs and leads to a redistribution of heat from the core of the body to the colder legs and to a fast decrease in core temperature. In contrast to general anaesthesia, thermoregulatory vasoconstriction in the arms persists (Fig. 8.1) [81].

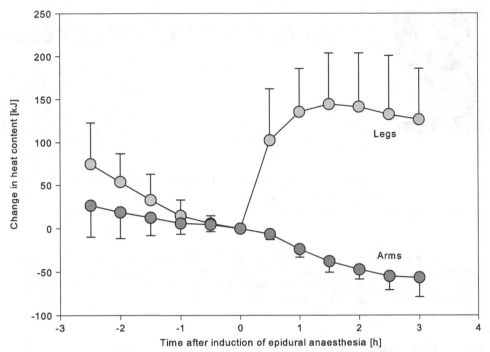

Fig. 8.1 Change in heat content of the arms and the legs in a volunteer experiment before and after induction of lumbal epidural anaesthesia. Before induction of epidural anaesthesia, the heat content of the arms and the legs decrease due to the cold exposure of the volunteers. After induction of epidural anaesthesia, the heat content of the legs increases due to the redistribution of heat from the core into the legs, whereas the heat content in the arms decreases further. The figure shows the mean values and standard deviation. (Drawn using data from [81].)

> This redistribution of heat is the most important factor in the drop in core temperature after induction of neuraxial anaesthesia, and persists throughout the following hours [81].

Linear phase

Comparable to general anaesthesia, core temperature then decreases linearly due to the thermal imbalance between heat production and heat loss (Fig. 8.2). The increased heat loss from the lower extremities also contributes to that thermal imbalance.

No active plateau phase

During general anaesthesia the linear phase ends with the re-emergence of autonomic thermoregulatory vasoconstriction and an active temperature plateau results. This is not possible during neuraxial anaesthesia because the nerve block will also block the triggered autonomic thermoregulatory vasoconstriction and shivering in the blocked regions [98]. In the unblocked regions, like the arms, autonomic thermoregulatory vasoconstriction and shivering is possible. However, upper-body shivering is relatively ineffective and often insufficient to prevent further hypothermia. In addition, thermoregulatory shivering is unpleasant and often necessitates antishivering treatment [112]. In contrast, a passive plateau can develop in well-insulated patients undergoing minor operations [98].

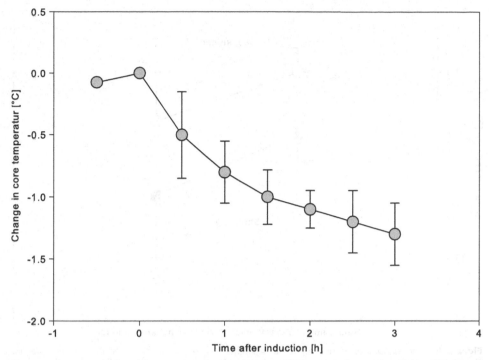

Fig. 8.2 Change in core temperature in a volunteer experiment before and after induction of lumbal epidural anaesthesia. The figure shows the mean values and standard deviation (Drawn using data from [81])

The influence of neuaxial anaesthesia on thermoregulation

In addition to the redistribution of heat and increased heat loss, neuraxial anaesthesia also impairs the autonomic control of thermoregulation. It seems that the hypothalamus incorrectly judges the peripheral temperature in the blocked area to be high. Before onset of regional anaesthesia the thermal input from that area indicated that the environment is cold. The afferent Aδ-fibres that transported the information from the cutaneous cold receptors to the hypothalamus fired tonically, whereas the afferent C-fibres transporting the information from the cutaneous warm receptors were nearly quiet. After blockade of both fibre types, the cutaneous temperature is no longer sensed as cold. This 'elevation' of skin temperature in the blocked area fools the hypothalamus and the autonomic thermoregulatory system into tolerating lower core temperatures without triggering a thermoregulatory response [98]. The thresholds for autonomic thermoregulatory vasoconstriction and shivering are reduced during neuraxial anaesthesia (Fig. 8.3) [98, 113, 114].

Perception of hypothermia during neuraxial anaesthesia

Although neuraxial anaesthesia typically causes hypothermia, patients often feel warmer after the induction of anaesthesia [98].

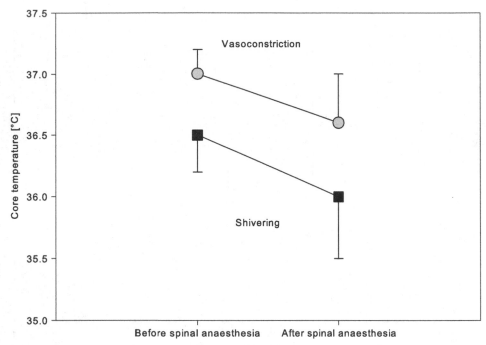

Fig. 8.3 Influence of spinal anaesthesia on the thermoregulatory thresholds of vasoconstriction and shivering. The figure shows the mean values and standard deviation. (Drawn using data from [114].)

This feeling of warmth is caused by the blockade of information from the cutaneous cold receptors to the brain. Therefore hypothermic patients under neuraxial anaesthesia often do not complain about feeling cold. However, when the neuraxial block resolves, the patients feel cold and often start to shiver [115].

Factors influencing the magnitude of hypothermia during neuraxial anaesthesia

The magnitude of the change in core temperature due to redistribution of heat can vary. The most important factor is the temperature of the peripheral tissues. The higher that temperature, the smaller the magnitude of redistribution. After a long exposure to a cold environment the peripheral tissues are cold, whereas after pre-warming of the patient the peripheral tissues are warmer. Therefore prewarming of the patient is an effective method to reduce the redistribution of heat during neuraxial anaesthesia [116]. The use of vasoconstrictors like phenylephrine during induction of neuraxial anaesthesia also reduces the magnitude of redistribution, comparable to the effect of vasoconstrictors during the introduction of general anaesthesia. The influence of neuraxial anaesthesia on the thermoregulatory thresholds is directly dependent on the height of the blockade. The higher the neuroaxial block, the larger the influence on the thermoregulatory threshold (Fig. 8.4) [117]. Extensive neuraxial blockades put the patients at a higher risk of hypothermia [115].

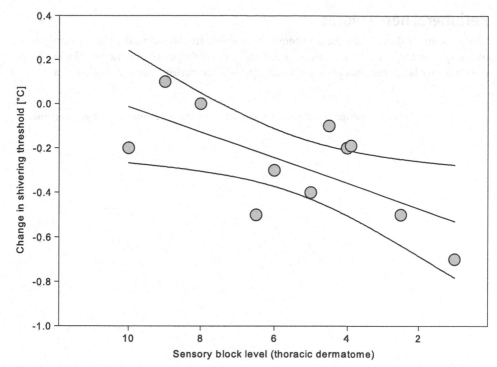

Fig. 8.4 Influence of spinal anaesthesia on the thermoregulatory thresholds of shivering in patients. (Drawn using data from [117]).

The thresholds for vasoconstriction and shivering are more reduced during neuraxial anaesthesia in older patients and this leads to a greater magnitude of hypothermia [115].

Spinal anaesthesia impairs autonomic thermoregulatory thresholds more than epidural anaesthesia because the sensory block is not so intense during epidural anaesthesia. The addition of a small dose of morphine to the local anaesthetic for spinal anaesthesia leads to lower core temperatures compared to spinal anaesthesia with local anaesthetic only. This may be caused by a cephalic spread of morphine in the cerebrospinal fluid to the hypothalamus.

Comparison of neuraxial anaesthesia and general anaesthesia

After neuraxial anaesthesia, mean core temperatures at admission to the postanaesthetic care unit of 34.4 to 35.9 °C have been described [118, 119], which is in the same range as core temperatures after general anaesthesia. The incidence of postoperative hypothermia has been described to be about 80%.

Several clinical studies have compared the influence of neuraxial anaesthesia and general anaesthesia on the incidence and magnitude of perioperative hypothermia. These studies indicate that the risk of perioperative hypothermia is comparable [118–120].

Peripheral nerve blocks

At the moment there is almost no literature available investigating the risk of perioperative hypothermia in patients undergoing surgery with peripheral nerve blocks. It is possible that large peripheral nerve blocks can induce perioperative hypothermia.

It is possible that large peripheral nerve blocks also can induce perioperative hypothermia.

Influence of regional anaesthesia and sedation

In this chapter the influence of regional anaesthesia with the additional use of sedation on the development of perioperative hypothermia is discussed.

Sedation is a well-established technique to improve patients acceptance and comfort during regional anaesthesia. It can be used before and during administration of regional anaesthesia to reduce pain at the puncture site, and to reduce fear and stress. Thereby sedation can improve cooperation of the patient and increase success rate, quality of the working conditions and work flow. During the surgical procedure sedation is often more convenient for the patient, the anaesthetist and the surgeon.

Sedation can range from minimal sedation and anxiolysis to deep analgosedation with an opioid or ketamine, and a hypnotic. Ideally the patient should be sedated to be relaxed, comfortable and cooperative during the procedure. Using conscious sedation, the patient's level of consciousness is depressed, but respiratory drive and airway reflexes are maintained and anaesthesia is provided by the local anaesthetic. A variety of drugs can be used to achieve these goals:

- Benzodiazepines
- Propofol
- Dexmedetomidine
- Remifentanil.

Benzodiazepines

Midazolam in particular is commonly used to reduce anxiety and to provide mild sedation during regional anaesthesia. Midazolam can cause a dose-dependent decrease in core temperature that is pronounced when sedation is more intense [72].

Sedation with midazolam can lead to a drop in core temperature.

Propofol

Propofol is another drug that is commonly used for sedation during regional anaesthesia [121]. Propofol also has a clear dose-dependent effect on the autonomic thermoregulatory thresholds [84] and can cause a dose-dependent decrease in core temperature by redistribution of heat, that can be clinically relevant [121].

Sedation with propofol can lead to a clinically relevant drop in core temperature.

Dexmedetomidine

Dexmedetomidine is a α2-adrenoreceptor agonist, like clonidine, with anxiolytic and dose-related sedative properties. Comparable to propofol, it also has a clear dose-dependent effect on the autonomic thermoregulatory thresholds (Fig. 9.1) [122]. Today, dexmedetomidine is not used routinely for sedation during regional anaesthesia.

Remifentanil

Remifentanil is often used for analgosedation during regional anaesthesia. It has a definite but relatively poor sedative effect. Data on its influence on autonomic thermoregulation are not available, but it can be assumed that it also has a dose-dependent effect on thermoregulation.

Comparison of neuraxial anaesthesia with sedation and general anaesthesia

Several studies have compared the influence of neuraxial anaesthesia with sedation and general anaesthesia on the incidence and magnitude of perioperative hypothermia. These studies indicate that the risk of perioperative hypothermia is comparable [123].

Comparison of neuraxial anaesthesia with sedation and neuraxial anaesthesia without sedation

In a prospective randomised trial, the influence of mild sedation with dexmedetomidine on the hypothermia rate during spinal anaesthesia was studied. There was no difference in the rate between sedated patients and the control group. In another trial, the influence of mild sedation with midazolam, ketamine or a combination of midazolam and ketamine or placebo was compared during spinal anaesthesia. There was no difference between the control group and the group that received sedation with midazolam. However, the group receiving ketamine had a slightly higher core temperature, whereas the group receiving ketamine and midazolam maintained their core temperature [112]. The authors discussed that this was probably because ketamine prevented the inhibition of the activated tonic thermoregulatory vasoconstriction that can be induced by midazolam [72], comparable to the effect of ketamine during induction of general anaesthesia [99]. Another possibility could be the stimulating effect of ketamine on energy expenditure.

The finding that the combination of regional anaesthesia and sedation does not seem to increase the hypothermia risk is a bit puzzling. Both regional anaesthesia and sedation have a risk of inducing hypothermia. Therefore it could be assumed that their combination would increase the risk of hypothermia. However, this is not the case. Maybe the stimulus for thermoregulatory vasoconstriction in the upper

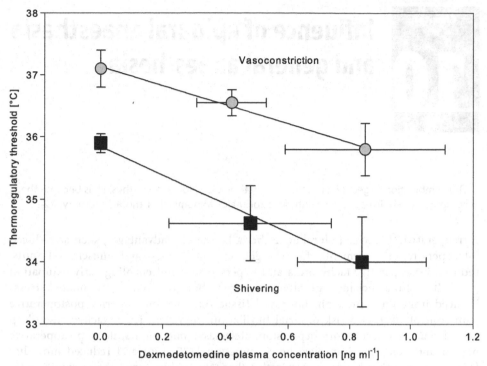

Fig. 9.1 Influence of increasing doses of dexmedetomidine on the thermoregulatory thresholds of vasoconstriction and shivering. The figure shows the mean values and standard deviation during mild and deep sedation. (Drawn using data from [122].)

extremities is so strong that mild sedation is unable to suppress it, or even more likely, the vasoconstriction in the upper extremities is so ineffective that the inhibition of it does not change anything [98].

The combination of regional anaesthesia and mild sedation does not increase the risk of hypothermia.

Chapter 10

Influence of epidural anaesthesia and general anaesthesia

The combination of general anaesthesia and thoracic epidural anaesthesia has become the technique of choice at many institutions for major abdominal or thoracic surgery [124].

Intraoperative thoracic epidural anaesthesia has several advantages, such as reduced intraoperative requirements for analgetics, anaesthetics and muscle relaxants, reduced intraoperative tachycardia and hypertension, and enabling early extubation [125]. It is also associated with attenuated stress hormone release, attenuated stress-induced immunosuppression, improved tissue oxygenation, superior postoperative pain control, decreased risk of atrial fibrillation, supraventricular tachycardia, deep vein thrombosis, respiratory depression, atelectasis, pneumonia, ileus, postoperative nausea and vomiting, improved bowel function [125, 126] and reduced mortality [126]. On the other hand, intraoperative thoracic epidural anaesthesia significantly increases the risk of intraoperative hypotension, pruritus, urinary retention, motor blockade [125, 126] and hypothermia [59, 92, 125, 127].

Epidural anaesthesia itself causes a drop in core temperature by vasodilatation and redistribution of heat from the core of the body to the legs [98], thermal imbalance between heat production and heat loss [110] and the influence on thermoregulatory thresholds [98]. Adding epidural anaesthesia to general anaesthesia further decreases the thermoregulatory thresholds and increases the rate of core cooling after induction of anaesthesia (Fig. 10.1)[92].

A nearly 1 °C lower core temperature at the end of the operation was also found in a large retrospective study with 433 patients undergoing radical prostatectomy, including retroperitoneal lymphadenectomy [125], where patients were anaesthetised with combined thoracic or lumbar epidural and general anaesthesia (Fig. 10.2).

In other studies, the differences between the treatment groups were smaller or non-existent. This was probably due to reduced doses of anaesthetics in the patients receiving general anaesthesia and epidural anaesthesia together with a sufficient intraoperative warming therapy. In contrast, in the study by Bito *et al.* [128], patients receiving general and epidural anaesthesia had higher core temperatures throughout surgery, although it is unclear why. Both patient groups were vasodilated during surgery and the authors discuss that a decreased cardiac output by thoracic sympathetic nerve blockade or the high temperature in the operating room of 25 °C may be responsible for this finding.

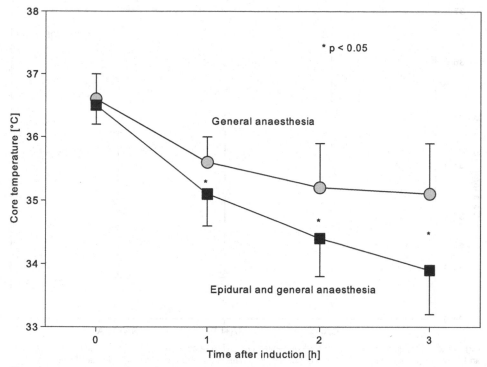

Fig. 10.1 Intraoperative core temperatures in patients receiving general or epidural and general anaesthesia during colorectal surgery. The figure shows the mean values and standard deviation. (Redrawn using data from [92].)

Why does the combination of epidural anaesthesia and general anaesthesia increase the risk of hypothermia?

There are several factors that are responsible for the increased risk of hypothermia during combined epidural and general anaesthesia.

1. In contrast to epidural anaesthesia alone, the combination of epidural and general anaesthesia also reduces the heat production of the body [98].
2. General anaesthesia and epidural anaesthesia together lead to pronounced vasodilation, thus enhancing redistribution of heat. This leads to a larger drop in core temperature compared to general anaesthesia alone.
3. The addition of epidural anaesthesia to general anaesthesia leads to higher skin temperature of the legs and therefore to a higher heat loss to the environment. This leads to a larger decrease in core temperature during the linear phase of the development of perioperative hypothermia.
4. General anaesthesia and epidural anaesthesia reduce both the vasoconstriction threshold. However, the epidural effect on thermoregulation is superimposed on the effect of general anaesthesia. As a result the vasoconstriction threshold is further reduced and vasoconstriction occurs at a lower core temperature [92].

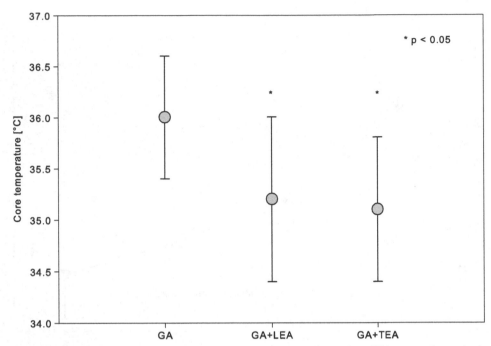

Fig. 10.2 Postoperative core temperatures in patients receiving general anaesthesia (GA) or general anaesthesia and lumbar epidural anaesthesia (GA+LEA) or general anaesthesia and thoracic epidural anaesthesia (GA+TEA) during radical prostatectomy including retroperitoneal lymphadenectomy. The figure shows the mean values and standard deviation, $p < 0.01$ vs. general anaesthesia. (Redrawn using data from [125].)

5. Under general anaesthesia alone, surgical stimulation may enhance the autonomic thermal responses [86] and lead to a higher vasoconstriction threshold during surgery. If surgical stimulation is blocked by the epidural anaesthesia this effect cannot occur.
6. Epidural anaesthesia prevents vasoconstriction in the legs. Typically, a mid-thoracic epidural block induces a thoracic, as well as a lumbar, sympathetic block when 8 to 10 ml of a local anaesthetic are used [92]. Therefore the lumbar sympathetic fibres responsible for thermoregulatory vasoconstriction in the legs are blocked.
7. If vasoconstriction is still initiated it is relatively ineffective, because it is restricted to the arms. Therefore, core temperature continues to decrease during combined epidural and general anaesthesia, whereas during general anaesthesia an active core temperature plateau occurs [98].

However, it should be stressed that patients with a combination of epidural and general anaesthesia can also be sufficiently warmed that they are normothermic [129].

The increased risk of perioperative hypothermia should not be an argument against combined epidural and general anaesthesia. As with all others, these patients need active perioperative warming management to maintain normothermia.

Influence of the surgical environment and surgery

In the previous chapters the tremendous importance of the anaesthetic procedures on the development of perioperative hypothermia was stressed. However, the surgical environment and procedures still have some influence.

Surgical environment

The influence of the cold surgical environment on the core temperature of anaesthetised animals was discovered nearly 100 years ago.

An experimental study as early as in 1924 found that normal dogs under general anaesthesia were only able to maintain their body temperatures at an environmental temperature near 31 °C. At lower room temperatures, the core temperatures of the dogs declined. However, the initial clinical data for patients in the 1950s did not confirm a low operating room temperature as a major problem for the development of perioperative hypothermia. In contrast, Clark *et al.* [130] described that operating room temperatures of more than 23.9 °C could cause significant increases in the core temperatures of adult surgical patients. In the 1960s it became clear that paediatric patients' core temperatures dropped during anaesthesia and the extent of core temperature drop could be related to cold operating room temperatures [8]. In the early 1970s, Morris and Kumar systematically studied the effects of operating room temperature on the development of perioperative hypothermia. They showed that the core temperature dropped reliably below 36 °C with operating room temperatures below 21 °C [131]. Operating room temperatures of more than 21 °C reduced the incidence and magnitude of hypothermia. During major vascular surgery [123], arthroplasties and liver resections, operating room temperatures of about 24 °C were associated with less hypothermia compared to lower operating room temperatures. In a recent study in patients undergoing orthopaedic surgery at operating room temperatures of nearly 26 °C only 10% of the patients became hypothermic [90].

Although none of these studies was a randomised controlled trial it seems to be clear that higher operating room temperatures are associated with less perioperative hypothermia. This is in accordance with the physics and physiology of heat exchange. From clinical trials, we do know that a typical mean skin temperature of an anaesthetised person is about 34 °C [86]. Calculating the heat loss from the skin to the environment for different room temperatures shows a linear relationship between cutaneous heat loss and room temperature (Fig. 11.1).

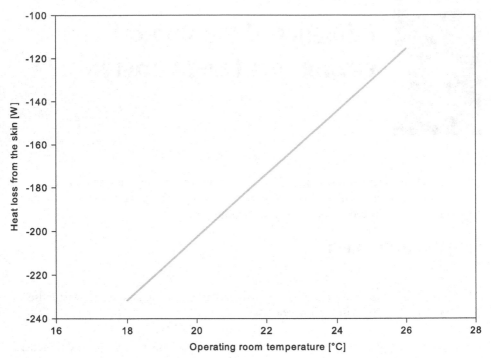

Fig. 11.1 Calculated heat losses from the skin by radiation and convection. The calculation is based on a mean skin temperature of 34 °C with an exposed body surface of 1.34 m^2 at different operating room temperatures.

As a rough estimate, an increase in room temperature of 1 °C reduces the cutaneous heat losses by about 10% and therefore elevation of operating room temperature is an effective measure to reduce the magnitude of hypothermia. In principle, the problem of perioperative hypothermia could be eliminated just by increasing the operating room temperature to 26–30 °C. However, high operating room temperatures do not provide adequate thermal comfort for surgeons, especially when wearing lead overalls and lead thyroid collars. Therefore the operating room temperature is always a compromise between working comfort for the surgical team and hypothermia prevention.

As a sensible compromise, the British NICE Guideline recommends that the ambient temperature in the operating room should be at least 21 °C, while the patient is exposed [17], the German and Austrian guideline recommends an operating room temperature of 21 °C [63] and the American ASPAN guideline recommends ambient room temperatures between 20 and 25 °C [18].

Surgical skin preparation

Another contributing factor for the development of perioperative hypothermia is the surgical skin preparation with disinfection solution. The patient is exposed to the cold environment and the skin is washed several times with the disinfectant. The surgical skin preparation solution is then warmed by the skin and evaporates. The calculated heat loss for the evaporation of water is 2.4 kJ g^{-1} and 1.1 kJ g^{-1} for ethanol [132]. Therefore the evaporation of 100 g of water would decrease the mean body temperature about 1 °C. However, the amount of surgical skin preparation solution used is typically lower than 100 ml, because a part of the solution remains on the swabs and is discarded. The amount of evaporation depends on the vapour pressure of the solution, on the scrubbing technique, and on the ambient temperature, humidity and air velocity in the operating room [132].

In a volunteer study, surgical skin preparation resulted in an increase in heat loss from about 80 W m^{-2} to 240–330 W m^{-2} in the first 5 minutes. However, after 15–20 minutes, the values returned to the baseline [132]. The calculated loss of the mean body temperature varied between 0.2 and 0.7 °C per m^2 of skin prepared, depending on the washing solution and the circumstances. However, even fairly large preparation areas of 45 cm × 45 cm represent an area of only 0.2 m^2 and result in a decrease in the mean body temperature of 0.04 to 0.14 °C [132].

> Although surgical skin preparation results in a short intense heat loss, the total impact on the mean body temperature and the perioperative heat balance is relative small for most surgical procedures. This may be different when very large areas are prepared, for example for off-pump coronary artery bypass surgery or in newborns and small children.

Heat loss from surgical incisions

To date it is difficult to determine precisely the contribution made by heat loss from the exposed wound to the total heat balance during surgery. Heat losses from the surgical field are mainly caused by the evaporation of water. The amount of water evaporated from the surgical incision depends on the size of the surgical field, on the exposed surface, and on the ambient temperature, humidity and air velocity in the operating room. In an animal and human study by Lamke *et al.* [133], evaporative water loss from wounds and exteriorised bowels was recording by the rate of increase of vapour concentration in a closed measuring chamber placed over the exposed abdominal cavity. In the animal experiment the evaporation of water from exteriorised bowels was initially 15 g h^{-1} and gradually decreased and stabilised at approximately 50% of the initial value after 20 min of exposure [133]. This would correspond to a heat loss of about 10 W initially and 5 W during the steady state conditions.

In the studied surgical patients the loss by evaporation from a minor incision with only slightly exposed viscera was about 2 g h^{-1} (corresponding to a heat loss of about 1.3 W), while during major exposure with exteriorised bowels, an evaporation of about 32 g h^{-1} was recorded, corresponding to a heat loss of 21 W. The authors concluded that the evaporative water loss from abdominal exposures is only of clinical importance during large and time-consuming procedures. These data were confirmed during orthopaedic surgery [134].

> The heat loss from the exposed wound ranges somewhat between 1 and 21 W and is less than often assumed.

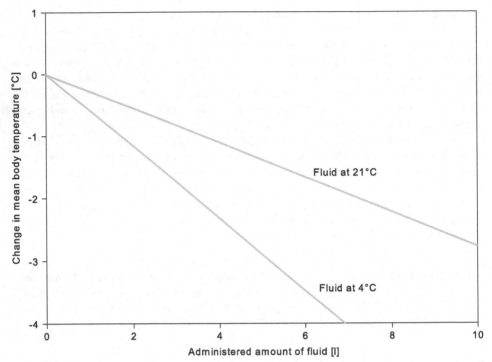

Fig. 11.2 Change in mean body temperature according to the quantity of administered fluid at different fluid temperatures. The calculation is based on the assumption of an undressed patient who weighs 70 kg with a metabolic rate of 93 W in a typical operating room with an operating room temperature of 21 °C. (Drawn and modified using data from [83].)

Irrigation, bleeding and infusion therapy

A last source of heat loss that is induced by surgery is the use of irrigation fluids and blood loss. Large amounts of irrigation fluids, for example during transurethral resection of the prostate can cause significant cooling of the patient [135]. Blood loss itself does not directly cause cooling. However, the replacement of the lost blood by unwarmed or inadequately warmed fluids causes hypothermia directly, depending on the amount of fluid and the temperature of the fluid given (Fig. 11.2).

Incidence of perioperative hypothermia

The first systematic studies about the incidence of perioperative hypothermia were conducted in the 1980s. In the study by Vaughan *et al.* [14] 60% of the 198 patients included had a core temperature of less than 36 °C and 13% were below 35 °C in the recovery room (Fig. 12.1). Elderly patients were particularly at risk of being hypothermic.

In a more recent study [59], published in 2003, the incidence of postoperative hypothermia after admission to the intensive care unit was 57.1%. In contrast to Vaughan's study [14], nearly 50% of the patients were warmed during the operation with forced-air warming devices. In several other studies published between 2005 and 2013 the incidence of postoperative hypothermia in intensive care units ranged between

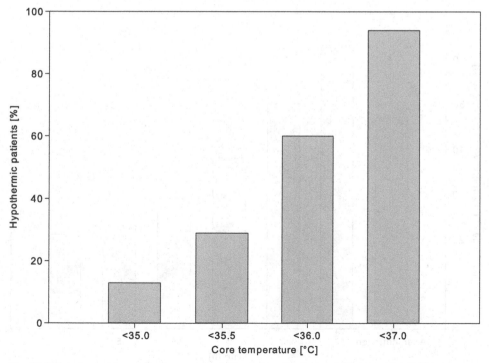

Fig. 12.1 Core temperatures of patients on admission to the recovery room. (Redrawn after [14].)

Table 12.1 Incidence of postoperative hypothermia

Publication date	Country	No. of patients	Surgery type	Actively warmed	Incidence of postoperative hypothermia	Ref.
2003	Thailand	184	General	48.9%	57.1%	[59]
2005	Portugal	185	Non-cardiac	43.8%	>75%	[58]
2008	Australia	171	Mixed	Not stated	48%	[137]
2009	Australia	5050	Mixed	Not stated	35%	[138]
2011	Australia and New Zealand	43.158	Cardiac	Not stated	66%	[141]
2013	Australia and New Zealand	50.689	Non-cardiac	Not stated	46%	[139]
2013	Netherlands	672	Orthopaedic	100%	29.6%	[136]
2015	US	58.814	Mixed	Virtually 100%	29.8%	[140]

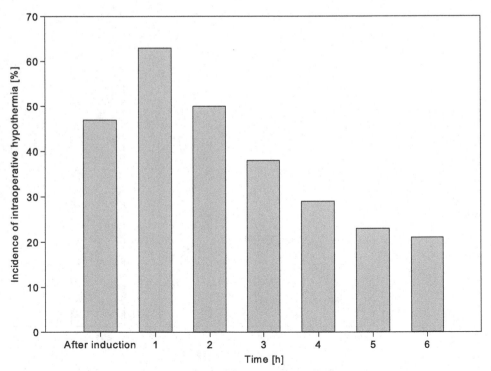

Fig. 12.2 Incidence of intraoperative hypothermia of 58 814 patients under active intraoperative warming therapy with forced-air warming. It can be seen that the incidence of hypothermia is time dependent, with the highest incidence occurring during the first few hours. (Redrawn using data from [140].)

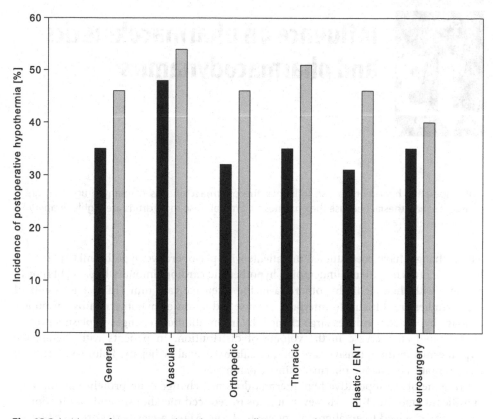

Fig. 12.3 Incidence of postoperative hypothermia in different types of surgery. The black columns represent data from [138], whereas the grey columns represent data from [139].

29.6 and >75%. [58, 136–139]. The largest of these studies included more than 50 000 patients [139] (see Table 12.1).

> Even nowadays, postoperative hypothermia is a significant clinical problem with a high incidence [139], despite all the possibilities for patient warming.

Due to effective intraoperative warming therapy, the core temperature of the patient typically reaches its nadir during the first hour of anaesthesia and then starts to rise again. Therefore the incidence of intraoperative hypothermia is higher than postoperative (Fig. 12.2) [140].

> In general there is no relevant difference in the postoperative hypothermia rate between the different types of surgery in a typical clinical setting (Fig. 12.3) [138–140].

Influence on pharmacokinetics and pharmacodynamics

13

> Perioperative hypothermia can influence the pharmacokinetics of many drugs that are used in anaesthesia, because the enzymes that metabolise most drugs are highly temperature sensitive [82].

These changes have been studied in patients with perioperative hypothermia [142, 143], but more often in patients undergoing hypothermic cardiopulmonary bypass [144] or in patients with therapeutic hypothermia in the intensive care unit [145]. The results of these studies are difficult to interpret, because induction of hypothermia by cardiopulmonary bypass also induces large changes by haemodilution, changes in plasma protein content and an increase in the volume of distribution. In patients with therapeutic hypothermia in the intensive care unit, circulatory, renal or hepatic failure and oedema can dramatically change pharmacokinetic parameters.

In general, perioperative hypothermia does not change drug protein binding by a significant amount [146]. However, it leads to reduced metabolism and elimination of drugs and can lead to an altered response to drugs. Many anaesthetics are metabolised in the liver by the cytochrome P450 enzyme system and the phase II enzymes, and are then eliminated through the kidneys. The cytochrome P450 enzyme system that is located either in the inner membrane of mitochondria or in the membrane of the endoplasmic reticulum of cells plays an important role in the activation and detoxification of many drugs. It consists of several isoforms that are abbreviated the following way: CYP as an abbreviation for cytochrome P450, followed by the number of the gene family, a letter indicating the subfamily and a final number for the individual gene. A typical example is CYP3A4.

The potential mechanisms by which hypothermia can alter drug metabolism are:

1. Hypothermia can change the configuration of the binding pocket of the enzyme, thereby decreasing the affinity of cytochrome P450 for specific drugs.
2. Hypothermia can reduce the affinity of oxygen for the ferric ion of the haem group in the cytochrome P450 enzyme system.
3. Hypothermia can decrease the rate of redox reactions of the enzyme system.
4. Hypothermia can change the activity of two cytochrome-P450-associated enzymes: nicotinamide adenine dinucleotide phosphate P450 reductase and cytochrome b5.
5. Hypothermia can change the fluidity of the lipid membrane in which the cytochrome P450 enzyme complex is embedded.
6. Hypothermia can reduce the activity of so-called phase II enzymes such as uridine 5′-diphospho-glucuronosyltransferase (UDP-glucuronosyltransferase). The phase II

enzymes are responsible for the process of glucuronidation of small hydrophobic molecules, thereby increasing blood solubility of the molecules to allow them to be eliminated by the kidneys [146].

7. Although passive filtration of substances in the glomeruli of the kidneys is not actively impaired by hypothermia, the energy-requiring tubular secretion of molecules is reduced [146].

Volatile anaesthetics

Hypothermia alters the pharmacokinetics of volatile anaesthetics because it increases their blood and tissue solubility (Fig. 13.1).

This means that at a given end-tidal concentration of a volatile anaesthetic, the blood and tissue anaesthetic content is higher in hypothermic patients than in normothermic patients. Therefore recovery from anaesthesia could be slower because larger amounts of the volatile anaesthetic need to be exhaled [82]. In addition, halothane, enflurane, isoflurane, sevoflurane and desflurane are metabolised in different amounts by cytochrome P450, mainly CYP2E1 in the liver. This metabolism is probably reduced by hypothermia. However, in a volunteer study, the washout rates of volatile anaesthetics were comparable between normothermic and hypothermic individuals [43] and the difference was minimal in a clinical trial.

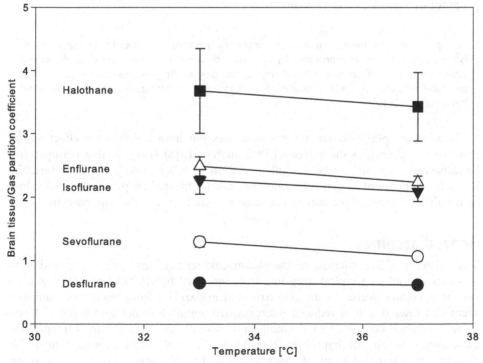

Fig. 13.1 Brain tissue/gas partition coefficients at 37 °C and 33 °C as a measure of tissue solubility for several volatile anaesthetics. (Drawn using data from [147].)

Perioperative hypothermia influences some pharmacokinetic parameters of volatile anaesthetics. Nevertheless, the clinical impact of these changes is minimal or negligible, especially with the newer agents like sevoflurane or desflurane.

Pharmacodynamics of volatile anaesthetics is also slightly changed by hypothermia. For example, the minimal alveolar concentration of isoflurane decreases by 5% per °C that the core temperature drops. However, this is not of great clinical importance.

Propofol

Propofol is commonly used as the hypnotic component of total intravenous anaesthesia and is metabolised by the CYP2B6 isoform and glucuronidated by UDP-glucuronosyltransferase. In a volunteer study, plasma concentrations of propofol were 28% higher in hypothermic volunteers at 34 °C compared to normothermic volunteers [148]. This difference was caused by a lower intercompartmental clearance of propofol and not by a change in the volume of distribution or a decrease in total body clearance, thus suggesting that hypothermia significantly alters the concentration present at the drug effect site. In contrast, a study in intensive care patients showed significantly lower total clearance of propofol in patients undergoing therapeutic hypothermia at 33–34 °C compared to a matched group of patients without hypothermia [145]. In the same patient population the plasma concentrations of propofol decreased during rewarming.

Perioperative hypothermia increases plasma concentrations of propofol. However, there is no study available showing that hypothermia delays extubation after propofol-based anaesthesia. Therefore, the clinical impact of this finding seems to be small, and propofol infusion regimens probably do not require adjustment in patients with mild hypothermia [149].

In addition, perioperative hypothermia does not have a significant effect on the processed EEG such as the bispectral EEG analysis (BIS) [149], so that perioperative hypothermia does not complicate interpretation of BIS values [149]. Therefore, the hypnotic component of general anaesthesia can be titrated by processed EEG values in mildly hypothermic patients in the same way as in normothermic patients.

Benzodiazepines

The influence of hypothermia on the pharmacokinetics of midazolam was studied in a volunteer trial as a typical drug that is metabolised by CYP3A4 and CYP3A5. As core temperature decreases, the elimination of midazolam from the central compartment decreases due to a reduced intercompartmental clearance and a reduced systemic clearance compared to normothermic volunteers. In intensive care patients undergoing therapeutic hypothermia at 33–34 °C, midazolam showed comparable clearance to a matched group of patients without hypothermia [145]. However, in the same patient population, the plasma concentrations of midazolam decreased during rewarming.

These data suggest that it is very unlikely that perioperative hypothermia delays recovery from anaesthesia due to its influence on the pharmacokinetics of midazolam given for premedication.

Opioids

Curiously, the influence of perioperative hypothermia on the pharmacokinetics of opioids has not been evaluated extensively, although residual amounts of opioids can delay postoperative recovery. Fentanyl, as an older opioid, is primarily metabolised in the liver by CYP3A4. In some animal and human studies plasma concentrations of fentanyl were higher during hypothermia [145]. This is probably caused by reduced distribution volume and reduced clearance. However, some of these data came from experiments with very high doses of fentanyl and very low core temperatures. Therefore, this may not be valid for normal doses of fentanyl and mild perioperative hypothermia.

There are some data about the influence of hypothermia on the pharmacokinetics of remifentanil from patients undergoing cardiac surgery with cardiopulmonary bypass. Remifentanil has a very short half-life due to rapid hydrolysis by non-specific blood and tissue esterases. In one study, hypothermia during cardiopulmonary bypass reduced elimination clearance by about 6% for each °C decrease in the core temperature [144]. This matches the results of a study with patients during rewarming from therapeutic hypothermia at 33–34 °C, where the plasma concentrations of remifentanil decreased during rewarming.

Perioperative hypothermia may increase the plasma concentrations of some opioids. However, the clinical impact of this finding is unclear.

Muscle relaxants

Muscle relaxants are commonly used during induction of general anaesthesia to facilitate tracheal intubation and are often used intraoperatively to improve surgical working conditions.

In contrast to volatile anaesthetics or midazolam, perioperative hypothermia markedly alters the pharmacokinetics of muscle relaxants.

The influence of perioperative hypothermia on the pharmacokinetics and pharmacodynamics of vecuronium [142], rocuronium [150] and atracurium [148] have been studied in detail.

Vecuronium

After injection of 0.1 mg kg^{-1} vecuronium, the duration of action until spontaneous recovery to a twitch tension of 10% is significantly increased by perioperative hypothermia [142]. In normothermic patients the duration of action was 28±4 min, whereas during hypothermia with a core temperature about 34.5 °C the duration of action was 62±8 min (Fig. 13.2).

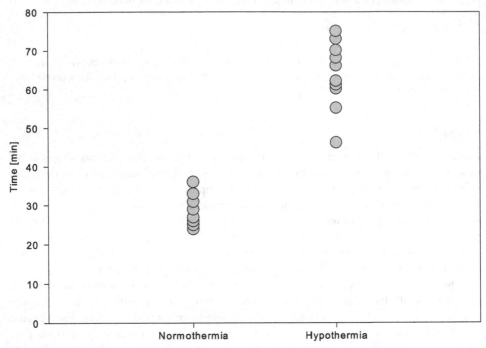

Fig. 13.2 Duration of action of 0.1 mg kg^{-1} vecuronium during normothermia and hypothermia with a core temperature of about 34.5 °C. Drawn using data from [142].

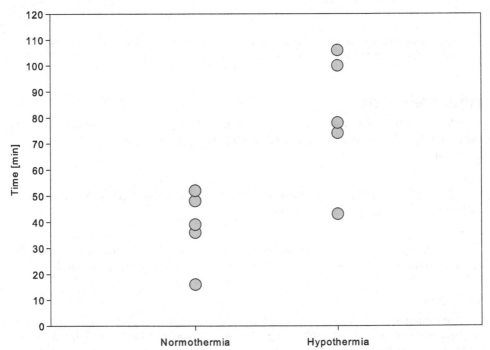

Fig. 13.3 Spontaneous recovery time with 0.1 mg kg^{-1} vecuronium from a twitch tension of 10% to a train-of-four ratio of 75% during normothermia and hypothermia with a core temperature of about 34.5 °C. (Drawn using data from [142].)

The corresponding times for spontaneous recovery from a twitch tension of 10% to a train-of-four ratio of 75% were 37±15 min during normothermia and 80±24 min during hypothermia.

There are several reasons for this increased duration of action and the slower recovery. The plasma clearance of vecuronium decreases during hypothermia by 11% per °C, as well as the rate constant for drug equilibration between plasma and effect site, which is slightly reduced by hypothermia.

Rocuronium

The newer neuromuscular blocker rocuronium also shows an increased duration of action and delayed recovery in hypothermic patients [150]. This is mainly caused by reduced plasma clearance of rocuronium during hypothermia. The volume of distribution is not different.

Atracurium

After injection of 0.5 mg kg^{-1} atracurium, the duration of action until spontaneous recovery to a twitch tension of 10% is significantly increased by perioperative hypothermia [148]. In normothermic volunteers, the duration of action was 44±4 min, whereas during hypothermia with a core temperature of about 34.5 °C, the duration of action was 68±7 min (about 60% longer). In contrast to vecuronium, the corresponding times for spontaneous recovery were not significantly altered. The reason for this difference remains unclear.

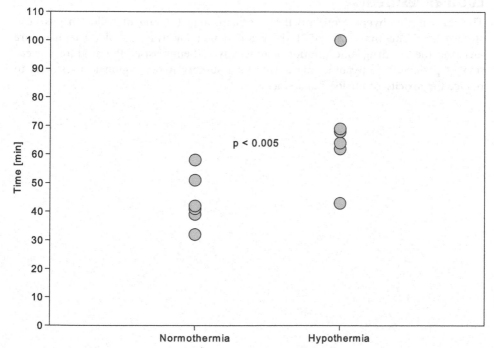

Fig. 13.4 Duration of action of 0.5 mg kg^{-1} atracurium during normothermia and hypothermia with a core temperature of about 34.5 °C. (Drawn using data from [148].)

Mivacurium

In vitro hydrolysis of mivacurium by pseudocholinesterase is not disturbed by mild hypothermia [151]. Clinical data are lacking.

Reversal of neuromuscular blockade

Residual effects of neuromuscular blockers may persist immediately after surgery, and even mild residual paresis can be associated with respiratory or pharyngeal muscle dysfunction in the postoperative recovery phase, leading to hypoxaemia and other pulmonary complications. The risk of residual effects of neuromuscular blockers increases when the duration of action and the recovery time is prolonged. In addition, hypothermia itself reduces muscle strength and may further aggravate muscle dysfunction. Reversal of neuromuscular blockade by neostigmine is not significantly delayed in hypothermic patients [142]. In hypothermic subjects, neostigmine has a lower volume of distribution, but the onset time of the maximum effect is slightly increased, probably because of reduced muscle blood flow to hypothermic muscles [143]. There is no change in the clearance, the maximum effect or duration of action of neostigmine in hypothermic subjects.

The recovery time to a train-of-four ratio of 0.9 after administration of sugammadex in patients with rocuronium-induced deep neuromuscular block is significantly prolonged in hypothermic patients. However, the difference was 125 seconds vs. 171 seconds and therefore not really relevant.

Local anaesthetics

The influence of hypothermia on the plasma protein binding of prilocain has been studied by Bachmann *et al.* [152]. They found that lowering the blood temperature increases the free drug concentration significantly and emphasised the need for prevention of perioperative hypothermia during long surgery under regional anaesthesia to reduce the toxicity of the local anaesthetic.

Influence on coagulation and blood loss

Perioperative hypothermia reduces platelet function and impairs the plasmatic coagulation cascade. This increases blood loss and increases transfusion requirements [153].

Physiology of blood coagulation

The coagulation system is a vital protective system of the body. It prevents blood loss by sealing sites of injured vessels and initiating wound healing. Nowadays the coagulation process is thought to occur mainly on specific cell surfaces. There are two types of cells involved: the tissue-factor-bearing cells of the subendothelium and the platelets.

Under normal conditions these two types of cells are separated by the endothelium, which forms a defence against thrombus formation until an injury of the vessel wall necessitates activation of coagulation. Once the vascular integrity breaches, the platelets and coagulation factors of the blood are exposed to the tissue-factor-bearing cells of the subendothelium, such as fibroblasts, pericytes and smooth vascular muscle cells, and the *initiation phase* of coagulation begins. Platelets adhere to subendothelial collagen directly or via interactions with the von Willebrand factor (vWF) that is released from endothelial cells after injury. At the same time, circulating activated factor VII (FVIIa) is bound to the tissue factor and trace amounts of thrombin are generated. Both processes lead to activation of platelets.

This is the start for the *amplification phase* of coagulation. The activated platelets change their shape via various signalling pathways, exposing membrane phospholipids to create a procoagulant surface. Additionally, the platelets release adenosine-diphosphate (ADP) and thromboxane A_2 (TXA_2), which further activate platelets in the vicinity. The trace amounts of thrombin generated in the initiation phase also activate coagulation factors on the platelet surface.

This processes results in the *propagation phase* of coagulation, occurring on the surface of the activated platelets. Large amounts of thrombin are generated via several complex mechanisms involving many coagulation factors, resulting in the cleavage of fibrinogen into fibrin monomers. These fibrin monomers are then polymerised by thrombin-activated factor XIII. The whole process is extremely complex and well regulated. However, it also depends on adequate environmental conditions like pH and temperature.

Influence of low temperature on blood coagulation

The function of cells and coagulation factors is influenced by low temperature. Hypothermia primarily seems to inhibit the initiation phase of coagulation.

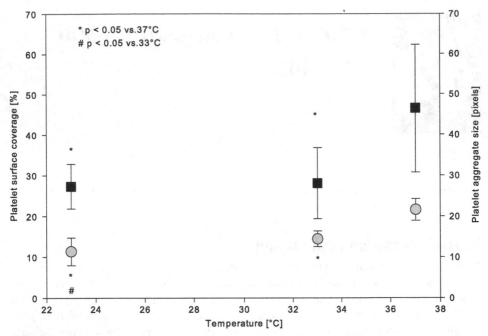

Fig. 14.1 Surface coverage of activated platelets as a parameter of platelet adhesion (grey circles) and the resulting platelet aggregation size (black squares) measured as a parameter of platelet aggregation at different temperatures. Both parameters decrease significantly with lower temperature. (Redrawn using data from [155].)

Endothelial cells

Endothelial cells release vWF from Weibel–Palade bodies after injury to help to form a carpet of platelets at the site of injury within seconds. These cells release significantly less vWF and slower at low temperature [154].

Platelets

Hypothermia also impairs platelet function in several ways. Adhesion of platelets to a surface, as well as aggregation of platelets is impaired (Fig. 14.1) [155]. Additionally, activation of platelets by vWF is inhibited by low temperature, leading to reduced production of thromboxane A_2 (Fig. 14.2) [156], which is essential for formation of the initial platelet plug.

Other ways of platelet activation, for example with adenosine diphosphate (ADP) or thrombin do not seem to be impaired by mild hypothermia.

As a result of all these changes in platelet functions, bleeding time as a simple clinical test of platelet function increases significantly and becomes clinically relevant with lowering skin temperature [156] or during hypothermia (Fig. 14.3).

Plasmatic coagulation

Hypothermia also impairs plasmatic coagulation. The rate of biochemical reactions is temperature dependent, with reduced rates at lower temperatures. This is also true for

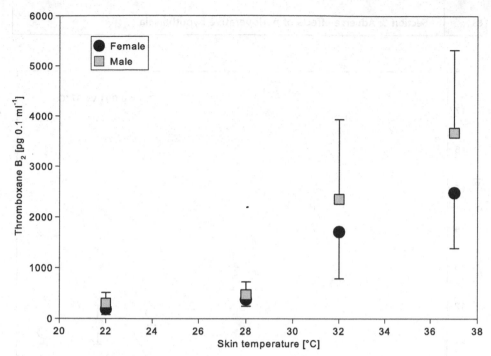

Fig. 14.2 Reduction of thromboxane B$_2$ concentration in shed blood at different skin temperatures. Thromboxane B$_2$ is the stable metabolite of thromboxane A$_2$ and is a parameter for the release of Thromboxane A$_2$ from activated platelets. It can be seen that the thromboxane B$_2$ concentration decreases steadily with lowering of the skin temperature. (Redrawn using data from [156].)

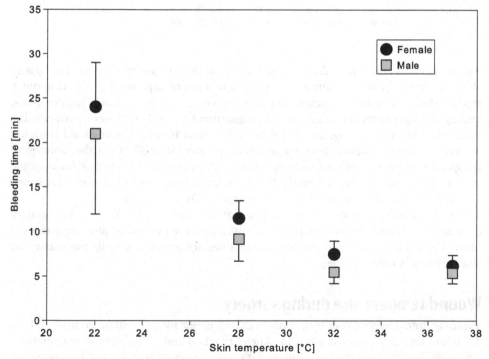

Fig. 14.3 Bleeding time after skin incision at different skin temperatures in male and female volunteers. It can be seen that the bleeding time increases steadily with lowering of the skin temperature from about 6 minutes up to more than 20 minutes. (Redrawn using data from [156].)

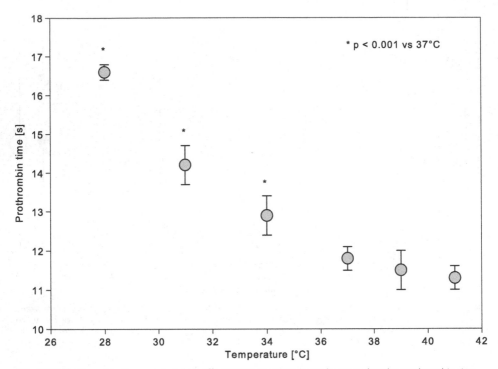

Fig. 14.4 Prothrombin time measured at different temperatures. It can be seen, that the prothrombin time increases steadily with lowering of temperature. (Redrawn using data from [157].)

the biochemical reaction of coagulation factors on the surface of platelets. The generation of thrombin on the surface is clearly temperature dependent [155]. Computer models show that thrombin generation is progressively delayed at lower temperatures, leading to longer clotting times in several coagulation tests [157, 158] when performed at these low temperatures (Fig. 14.4). However, this effect is often unrecognised clinically because all the coagulation tests are normally performed at 37 °C in the laboratory, irrespective of the patient's actual temperature. When these *in vitro* tests – for example prothrombin time or activated partial thromboplastin time (Fig. 14.5) – are performed at lower temperatures the impairment is obvious [153].

The impairment can also be seen in point-of-care methods like thrombelastography or rotational thrombelastometry [158] when the tests are performed at lower temperatures. The clotting times and clot formation times are prolonged, while the maximum clot firmness is reduced [158].

Wound temperature during surgery

Typically, intraoperative core temperatures during major surgery seldom go below 34 °C. Therefore the relevance of changes in platelet function and coagulation at temperatures below 30 °C may be questioned. However, it must be stressed that it is not core temperature that is responsible for coagulation. It is the wound temperature that is decisive because that is the place where blood loss and coagulation takes place and wound temperatures are

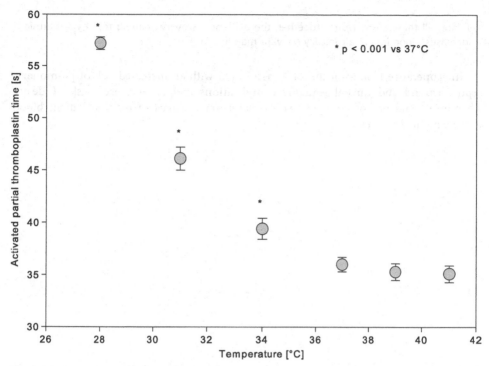

Fig. 14.5 Activated partial thromboplastin time measured at different temperatures. The activated partial thromboplastin time increases steadily with lowering of temperature. (Redrawn using data from [157].)

typically below the core temperature. Wound temperatures with regard to perioperative hypothermia have been measured only sparsely. The thoracic wound temperature after sternotomy is about 32.5 °C [159]. Similar temperatures have been measured in animals during abdominal surgery [133, 160]. In humans, bowel surface temperatures range between 26 and 35 °C [133, 161], and wound temperature is about 31.5±1.5°C during orthopaedic back surgery [134]. Sufficient prewarming [79, 162] or intraoperative warming increases peripheral skin and tissue temperature [163] and therefore can increase wound temperature. However, there is no clear linear relationship between core temperature and wound temperature [133, 161].

Influence of perioperative hypothermia on blood loss and transfusion requirement

Various studies have reported that mild hypothermia influences intra- and postoperative blood loss and transfusion requirement [153]. Most studies have reported that hypothermia increases blood loss [164–169], although some have found no difference [170] or even that hypothermia reduces blood loss. In the meta-analysis of published, randomised, controlled trials [153] the average blood loss was approximately 16% higher in hypothermic patients. In the same meta-analysis the relative risk for transfusion was approximately 22% higher in the hypothermic patients [153].

Taking all these study results together, the evidence is overwhelming that hypothermia increases blood loss at a clinically relevant magnitude.

Intraoperative blood transfusion is associated with an increased risk of pulmonary, septic, wound and thromboembolic complications and an increased risk of death. Therefore avoidance of perioperative hypothermia is a part of modern patient blood management strategies.

Adverse effects of perioperative hypothermia

Feeling cold and shivering

> Perioperative hypothermia causes substantial postoperative thermal discomfort [171] and about 50% of patients remember shivering and a feeling of intense cold as the most distressing memory of their anaesthetic management.

The intense feeling of being cold can last for more than 1 hour if the patients are not actively warmed (Fig. 15.1) [171].

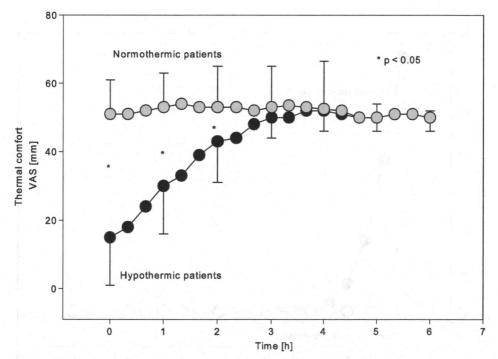

Fig. 15.1 Thermal discomfort of hypothermic patients after colon surgery lasts for several hours compared to normothermic patients. The thermal comfort was analysed using a 100 mm visual analogue scale (VAS) with 0 mm indicating intense cold and 50 mm indicating thermal comfort. (Redrawn using data from [171].)

Shivering

Shivering is common in the early postoperative period. It is often a consequence of perioperative hypothermia, but it is important to know that hypothermia is not the only possible reason. In general, shivering can be divided in thermoregulatory shivering and non-thermoregulatory shivering.

Postoperative shivering occurs frequently (up to 60%) [37] in the postanaesthetic care unit (Fig. 15.2). Without active warming, postoperative shivering can be present throughout the first hour after anaesthesia.

Thermoregulatory shivering

Most postoperative shivering is thermoregulatory shivering [37, 172] and occurs when anaesthetic-induced thermoregulatory inhibition disappears and the thermoregulatory threshold for shivering threshold returns to normal [37]. This can be caused by persistent perioperative hypothermia, but may also be caused by an elevation of the core temperature set-point and the thermoregulatory thresholds, for example by fever [37, 172] or an inflammatory response to surgery [62], especially after operations on infected tissues [172].

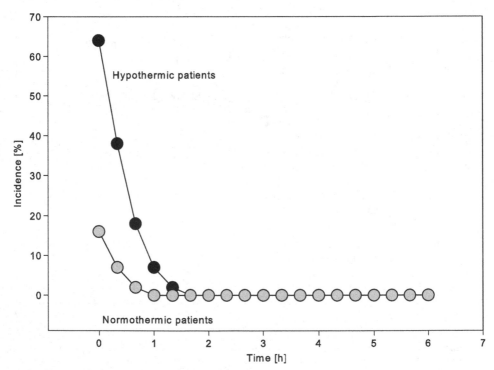

Fig. 15.2 Incidence of postoperative shivering of hypothermic and normothermic patients after colon surgery. (Redrawn using data from [171].)

Non-thermoregulatory shivering

Non-thermoregulatory shivering is also called shivering-like tremor [37]. The aetiology of non-thermoregulatory shivering is poorly understood. It can occur after anaesthesia with volatile anaesthetics [173] or after the administration of remifentanil. It is also associated with postoperative pain [37, 174], young age and endoprosthetic surgery.

Differentiation between thermoregulatory and non-thermoregulatory shivering

Typically patients with perioperative hypothermia and thermoregulatory shivering have a lower postoperative core temperature compared with their individual preoperative value. They are almost always significantly vasoconstricted, which means that the temperature of the fingertips is lower than the temperature of the forearm. Additionally, the patients often feel cold [172]. Patients with postoperative fever and thermoregulatory shivering have a higher postoperative core temperature compared with their individual preoperative value. These patients are also vasoconstricted and feel cold.

In contrast, patients with non-thermoregulatory shivering are usually normothermic and vasodilated with a temperature at fingertips equal to the temperature of the forearm. Additionally, the patients do not feel cold.

> In clinical practice, the presence of a significant forearm–fingertip temperature gradient can be estimated by simply touching the skin of the forearm at the radial side of the arm midway between the wrist and the elbow, and the fingertip of the index finger opposite the nail bed.

Efficacy of shivering for rewarming

Shivering is not an effective method of rewarming, because it also increases heat loss and therefore does not speed up the rewarming process.

Oxygen uptake and haemodynamic changes during shivering

> Shivering increases the work and oxygen demand of the skeletal muscles. This demand is met by an increase in oxygen uptake and cardiac output. In most patients, arterial blood pressure and heart rate are not changed significantly [42, 171], but systemic vascular resistance decreases and oxygen extraction from the blood increases [42] (Fig. 15.3).

Vigorous shivering increases metabolic heat production and oxygen uptake [37, 42]. In 1966, Roe et al. [15] had already described that patients with a low intraoperative core temperature had an increase in oxygen consumption after surgery. Patients with a minimal drop in core temperature had an increase in oxygen consumption of about 5%, whereas patients with a larger drop in core temperature had an increase in oxygen consumption of 92%. Interestingly, the patients with the largest drop in core temperature were the oldest patients and developed an increase in oxygen consumption of only about 40% [15].

Based on the results of some of these studies, many anaesthesiologists believed that postoperative shivering dramatically increases total body oxygen consumption up to more

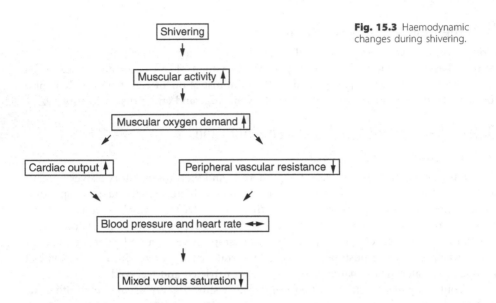

Fig. 15.3 Haemodynamic changes during shivering.

than 730% above baseline. They were afraid that this massive increase in oxygen consumption would lead to cardiac complications like myocardial ischemia or arrhythmia. However, patients with extremely high values of oxygen consumption were generally relatively young and healthy, and these values were only measured during short periods of shivering. Recent studies in older patients have confirmed the results of Roe *et al.* [15] that shivering increases oxygen consumption by only about 40% [175]. In recent years it has become clear that shivering – in contrast to perioperative hypothermia – is not associated with cardiac complications [167, 175, 176]. However, postoperative shivering can be associated with mild hypoxaemia.

Pain during shivering

Shivering may aggravate postoperative pain by movement and stretching surgical incisions in individual patients [37]. However, in general, postoperative pain is similar in patients with and without shivering [175].

Failure of monitoring devices during shivering

During intense shivering, ECG signals are often disturbed. These artefacts can be used to determine shivering [174], but more often these artefacts cause unnecessary alarms and sometimes mimic significant arrhythmia.

Motion artefacts during shivering can hinder adequate measurement of oxygen saturation with pulse oximetry and can cause incorrect values for heart rate and oxygen saturation. Additionally, shivering can cause significant malfunction time without any value for oxygen saturation. Although the technology of these devices has improved since these studies, this phenomenon can still be observed and may be important, because during shivering mild oxygen desaturation can occur. Shivering can also disturb non-invasive blood pressure measurements with automatic devices leading to significant malfunction time and alarms. Shivering may also disturb invasive blood pressure measurement by motion artefacts.

Intensive shivering can disturb the ECG, and monitoring of oxygen saturation and blood pressure measurement.

Other adverse events during shivering

It has been reported that severe shivering can increase intracerebral [177] and intraocular pressure [177], which is undesirable after surgery in these areas. Extreme shivering has also been reported to lead to wound dehiscence [177]. However, such adverse events have only been reported anecdotally and do not play a significant role.

In general, shivering is not an effective method for rewarming, but is associated with several important and unpleasant side effects. Therefore treatment of postoperative shivering is appropriate [37].

Postoperative pain, pulmonary complications and length of stay in the postanaesthetic care unit

Postoperative pain

It can be assumed that thermoregulatory shivering may aggravate postoperative pain by movement and stretching surgical incisions in individual patients [37]. Several studies have tried to find out if patients that develop perioperative hypothermia have more postoperative pain beyond the phase of shivering. In studies with patients undergoing orthopaedic surgery, no differences in postoperative pain scores between the actively warmed patients and the control patients were found, but in one study the hypothermic patients required more opioids. In studies with patients undergoing abdominal or abdominal, thoracic, or vascular surgery there were no differences in postoperative analgesic requirements [167, 168, 178] or pain intensity [167, 178, 179] between normothermic and hypothermic patients. The same was true for outpatients [180].

In a typical clinical setting, postoperative pain and analgesic requirements do not seem to be affected by mild postoperative hypothermia.

Pulmonary complications

Mild perioperative hypothermia can lead to a significantly higher incidence of postoperative mild hypoxaemia in the postanaesthetic care unit, even when the patients receive supplemental oxygen [176]. This can be observed especially during postoperative shivering, but is not only associated with shivering and may be caused by higher oxygen consumption during shivering or increased pulmonary shunting. In animals it was shown that hypothermia inhibits hypoxic pulmonary vasoconstriction significantly. In addition, in patients recovering from intraoperative hypothermia the alveolar–arterial difference in oxygen tension ($AaDO_2$) is higher during hypothermia.

Mild perioperative hypothermia can lead to a significantly higher incidence of postoperative mild hypoxaemia in the postanaesthetic care unit. The hypothermia-induced changes in pulmonary function (inhibited hypoxic pulmonary vasoconstriction, higher $AaDO_2$) and residual effects of muscle relaxants increase the risk of hypothermic patients needing reintubation after planned extubation [181].

Prolonged length of stay in the postanaesthetic care unit

In a prospective randomised trial with adult patients undergoing major abdominal surgery, hypothermic patients required a significantly longer time to reach fitness for discharge, using a modified Aldrete and Kroulik scoring system to assess fitness for discharge. The normothermic patients needed 53±36 minutes, whereas the hypothermic patients needed 94 ±65 minutes. When a core temperature of more than 36 °C was used as additional criterion, the times were 66±46 minutes and 159±57 minutes, respectively [178]. Similar results were obtained after abdominal surgery [166], in patients after open radical prostatectomy, after total hip arthroplasty or in outpatients. However, other studies could not find a difference in the recovery time between warmed and unwarmed patients [180]. Surprisingly, in infants and children, mild perioperative hypothermia also did not prolong postanaesthetic recovery [182, 183].

These different results may be explained by differences in the patient groups and the methodology. In the clinical setting, consciousness, respiratory function, circulatory function, renal function, and nausea and vomiting are not the only discharge criteria. Adequate control of postoperative pain is also a very important criterion for discharging a patient. Therefore, very often patients stay in the recovery room even if the Aldrete and Kroulik score suggests that the patient is fit for discharge.

Hypothermic patients after major surgery need a longer time to be fit for discharge compared to normothermic patients.

Cardiovascular consequences

Cardiac events like myocardial infarction, congestive heart failure, myocardial ischaemia and rhythm disturbances are the leading cause of death during and immediately after anaesthesia. Perioperative hypothermia is known to increase the risk of myocardial ischaemia [176], morbid cardiac events (like unstable angina, myocardial infarction or cardiac arrest) [167] and ventricular tachycardia [167] in patients with coronary heart disease or at risk of coronary heart disease. These events mainly occur more than 6 hours after surgery [3] and therefore are usually not visible for anaesthesiologists.

The pathophysiology of these events is more complex than initially thought. For several years it was suspected that especially postoperative shivering, with its associated massive increase in oxygen consumption, was responsible. In the last 15 years it has become clear that this is not true, because the threshold for thermoregulatory shivering is very low in elderly patients [65, 175] and these high-risk patients rarely shiver. More importantly, perioperative myocardial ischemia is unrelated to shivering [167, 175]. Therefore, shivering does not directly lead to myocardial ischaemia or infarction [82]. It is more likely that the cardiac events are mediated by adrenergic responses that are triggered by hypothermia.

Adrenergic responses triggered by hypothermia in volunteers

Thermoregulatory vasoconstriction appears when the body is exposed to a cold environment and reduces skin perfusion in the acra by release of norepinephrine from sympathetic nerves at the arteriovenous shunts [38]. In volunteers with even very mild hypothermia, the plasma norepinephrine concentrations rise significantly more than 200% as a consequence of thermoregulatory vasoconstriction (Fig. 17.1) [65, 184–186]. Hypothermia also evokes adrenomedullary activation with a significant release of epinephrine from the adrenals when the core temperature drops about 1 °C below the baseline [184–186], which is normally above the threshold for thermoregulatory shivering.

Haemodynamic consequences of hypothermia in volunteers

During induction of very mild hypothermia, peripheral vasoconstriction increases mean arterial blood pressure by about 15 to 20% [185] without increasing the heart rate [185]. When the core temperature drops about 1 °C below the baseline, the release of plasma epinephrine leads to an increase in heart rate and cardiac output [185]. However, in healthy volunteers these haemodynamic changes do not lead to coronary vasoconstriction. Myocardial perfusion increases in a manner that matches myocardial oxygen consumption [186].

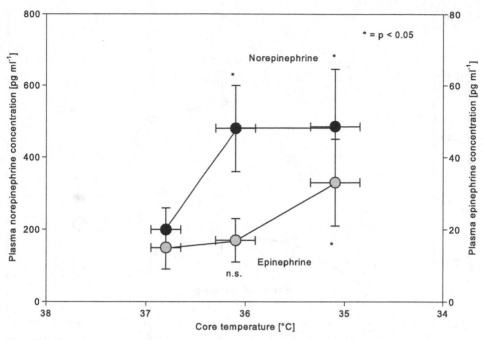

Fig. 17.1 Change in plasma catecholamine concentrations during induction of hypothermia in volunteers. During very mild hypothermia only the concentration of norepinephrine rises. When the core temperature drops about 1 °C below the baseline, plasma epinephrine concentration also starts to rise. The asterisks mark significant changes compared to baseline ($p < 0.05$). (Redrawn using data from [185].)

In addition, perioperative hypothermia reduces baroreflex function, which is an important short-term control system for maintaining cardiovascular stability during haemodynamic challenges. This system is already impaired by many anaesthetics (e.g. volatile anaesthetics, propofol), but hypothermia further reduces its function during anaesthesia and several hours after anaesthesia. Heart rate variability is also influenced by hypothermia. However, it is unclear if this finding has any clinical importance for cardiovascular morbidity that is induced by perioperative hypothermia.

Hypothermia increases blood viscosity. A decrease in temperature of 1 °C increases plasma viscosity by roughly 2–3%. However, in the perioperative setting the effects of changes in haematocrit or fibrinogen levels are much more important compared to the effect of hypothermia.

Adrenergic responses, haemodynamic and cardiac consequences of hypothermia in patients

In surgical patients, adrenergic responses triggered by hypothermia are also visible. Hypothermic patients have postoperatively significant higher plasma concentrations of norepinephrine [179] compared to normothermic patients (Fig. 17.2). The epinephrine levels increased compared to the preoperative values but there was no significant difference between the hypothermic and the normothermic patient groups (Fig. 17.3) [179].

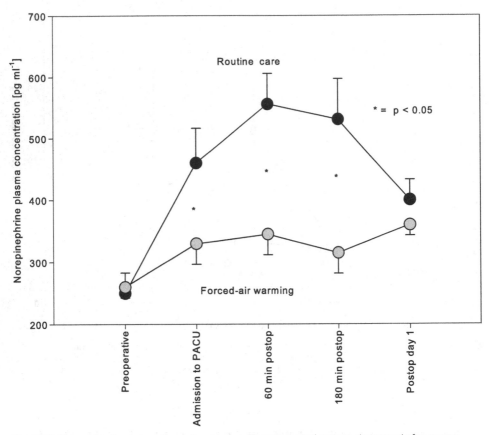

Fig. 17.2 Change in plasma norepinephrine concentrations in surgical patients during and after surgery. During and after the operation, plasma norepinephrine concentrations rise in both groups, but the increase in the unwarmed group is significantly larger. The asterisks mark significant differences between the two patient groups ($p < 0.05$). (Redrawn using data from [179].)

As a consequence, postoperative blood pressure is higher in hypothermic patients [167, 179]. However, in patients with risk of coronary heart disease, perioperative hypothermia is associated with myocardial ischaemia and morbid cardiac events. In 1993 Frank *et al.* [176] observed that patients developing perioperative hypothermia with a core temperature below 35 °C have a higher rate of myocardial ischaemia during and after surgery. In 1997 he proved, in a large randomised controlled trial, that perioperative hypothermia is associated not only with ECG changes, but also with relevant morbid cardiac events like unstable angina, myocardial infarction, arrhythmia and cardiac arrest [167]. Also in large retrospective studies, more myocardial infarctions [187] and other cardiovascular complications [187, 188] could be observed in hypothermic patients. Many of these cardiac events are linked to myocardial ischaemia or myocardial infarction. In general perioperative myocardial infarction can be divided into two distinct types [189]. Perioperative myocardial infarction type I is caused by an unstable coronary plaque. Sympathetic hyperactivity with increased concentration of plasma catecholamines, haemodynamic instability and coronary vasoconstriction leads to plaque erosion or rupture thus leading to acute coronary thrombosis (Fig. 17.4) [189].

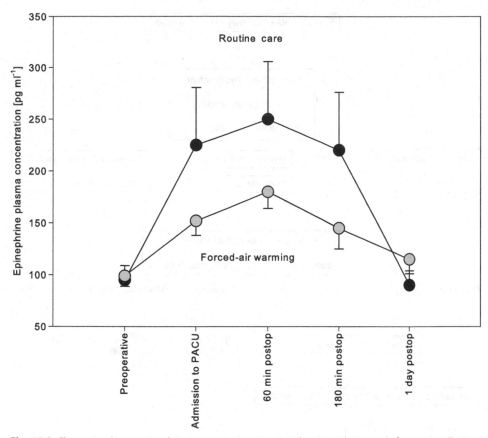

Fig. 17.3 Change in plasma epinephrine concentrations in surgical patients during and after surgery. During and after the operation, plasma epinephrine concentrations rise in both groups. The increase in the unwarmed group is larger, but this difference is not significant. (Redrawn using data from [179].)

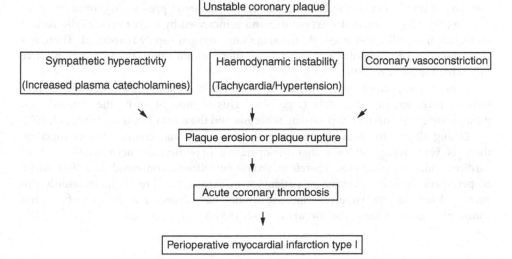

Fig. 17.4 Pathophysiology of perioperative myocardial infarction type I. (Modified and simplified after [189].)

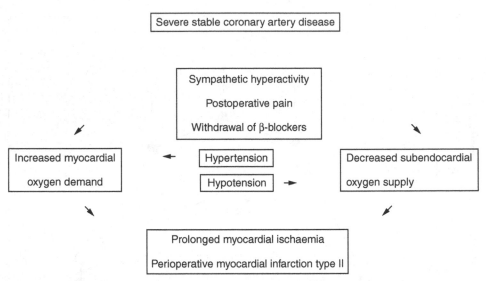

Fig. 17.5 Pathophysiology of perioperative myocardial infarction type II. (Modified and simplified after [189].)

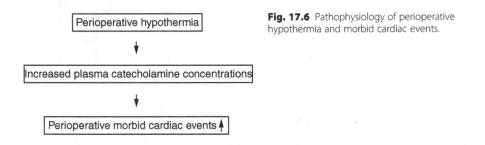

Fig. 17.6 Pathophysiology of perioperative hypothermia and morbid cardiac events.

The more frequent perioperative myocardial infarction type II is caused by a myocardial oxygen supply–demand imbalance in patients with severe pre-existing coronary artery disease (Fig. 17.5). Myocardial oxygen demand is increased by heart rate, arrhythmia and increased myocardial wall stress. At the same time, oxygen supply is reduced. There is a wide spectrum of myocardial ischaemia, from silent, minor injury to overt perioperative myocardial infarction [189].

In both types, sympathetic hyperactivity with elevated plasma catecholamine concentrations plays an important role (Fig. 17.6). This is thought to be the link between perioperative hypothermia, myocardial ischaemia and the morbid cardiac events [82, 167].

Taking all this information on the pathophysiology and clinical studies together, there is very strong evidence that perioperative hypothermia increases the risk of cardiovascular complications. Therefore, several guidelines recommend the maintenance of perioperative normothermia in patients with cardiac risk [16, 190]. In addition to increased cardiac risk, large retrospective studies have found that the risk of cerebral transient ischemic attack [188] or stroke [187, 188] is also increased.

Influence on wound healing and infections

Despite strict asepsis, postoperative wound infection is a common and serious complication of surgery [191], associated with enormous costs [17]. Maintenance of perioperative normothermia can reduce the number of postoperative wound infections significantly [168, 192].

Postoperative wound infections after surgery are a common and serious complication that increases postoperative morbidity of the patients and the associated costs considerably [17, 168, 193]. They can be detected five to nine days after surgery and therefore are usually not visible for anaesthesiologists.

Physiology of wound healing

Wound healing is a very complex process that involves blood cells, parenchymal cells, extracellular matrix and several mediators and cytokines. Immediately after injury, blood vessels constrict and coagulation starts. Platelets adhere and aggregate and release the content of their granules to form a clot together with coagulation factors. Several mediators and cytokines are released causing *inflammation*. Growth factors evoke chemotaxis of neutrophils, monocytes and fibroblasts and these cells release additional cytokines. Several hours after injury *re-epithelisation* of the wound begins and formation of granulation tissue starts. After a few days the last phase of wound healing begins with *wound contraction* and *extracellular matrix reorganisation*.

This complex process of wound healing is disturbed by infection. During surgery, every wound is contaminated with bacteria. The first hours after bacterial contamination constitute a decisive period during which wound infection is either established or not [193]. The effects of antibiotic prophylaxis, hypothermia and hypoperfusion are especially important during this decisive period [193].

Influence of low temperatures on the physiology of wound healing

Hypothermia impairs wound healing and immune function in several ways. Perioperative hypothermia induces thermoregulatory vasoconstriction and thereby decreases subcutaneous tissue perfusion which, in turn, decreases tissue oxygenation [194]. Reduced tissue oxygenation clearly increases the risk of wound infections [195]. The effect of thermoregulatory vasoconstriction on tissue oxygenation can be modified by local cooling or warming [194], which means that local warming, even in hypothermic subjects, can increase tissue oxygenation.

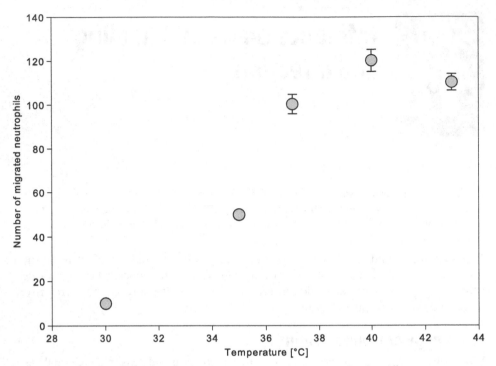

Fig. 18.1 Average number of migrated neutrophils ± SEM by chemotaxis to *E. coli* at different temperatures. (Redrawn using data from [196].)

Additionally, the initial defence against bacteria relies very much on local recruitment and function of leukocytes. Chemotaxis of neutrophils to bacteria is dramatically reduced at lower temperatures (Fig. 18.1) [196], as well as phagocytosis and oxidative killing of bacteria (Figs. 18.2 and 18.3) [197].

Perioperative hypothermia also suppresses various subpopulations of lymphocytes and decreases the production of several substances, such as interleukin-2 (IL-2), which plays an important role in immune response. IL-2 is a growth factor for T-lymphocytes and stimulates production of interferon-γ, tumour necrosis factor-α (TNF-α) and IL-4, IL-5 and IL-6, which in turn accelerate inflammation [198]. Hypothermia also reduces production of IL-1-β [198], which induces angiogenesis and activation of fibroblasts, and negatively influences monocyte function, which can also be linked to infection complications after surgery [199]. Additionally, wound healing is slower in hypothermic tissue. Collagen deposition near the wound is reduced in hypothermic patients [168], which may facilitate bacterial spread (Fig. 18.4).

Animal experiments

In animal experiments, resistance to dermal infection with *Staphylococcus aureus* or *Eschericha coli* was reduced under hypothermic conditions. It could also be shown that perioperative hypothermia has detrimental effects on healing of colonic anastomosis and that restoring normothermia after anaesthesia improved survival of sepsis. However, the last effects have not been shown in humans yet.

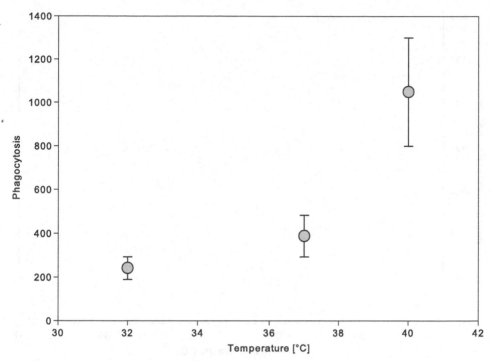

Fig. 18.2 Average phagocytosis capacity of neutrophil granulocytes measured in fluorescence units ± standard deviation at different temperatures. (Redrawn using data from [197].)

Influence of perioperative hypothermia on wound healing in clinical studies

In 1996 the first and most important clinical study on the influence of hypothermia on wound infection was published by Kurz *et al.* [168]. In this study, entitled 'Perioperative normothermia to reduce the incidence of surgical-wound infection and shorten hospitalisation', patients undergoing colorectal surgery were randomised to routine intraoperative thermal care or to active warming with forced-air and infusion warming. It was planned to study a maximum of 400 patients, but the study was stopped after 200 patients were enrolled, because the incidence of surgical-wound infections in the two study groups differed significantly. As intended, core temperatures were significantly lower in the group of patients with routine intraoperative thermal care (34.7±0.6 °C) than in the active warming group (36.6±0.5 °C) and remained significantly lower for several hours postoperatively. Intraoperative vasoconstriction was observed very frequently (74%) in the patients assigned to routine intraoperative thermal care, but only in 6% of those assigned to active warming. The same was observed for postoperative vasoconstriction (78 vs. 22%).

Wound infections were found in 18 of 96 (19%) patients treated with routine intraoperative thermal care, but in only 6 of 104 (6%) of patients assigned to active warming. This means that wound infections were reduced to one-third by active warming, and this is highly significant. Additionally, the sutures in the routine intraoperative thermal care group were removed one day later compared to the patients in the active warming group,

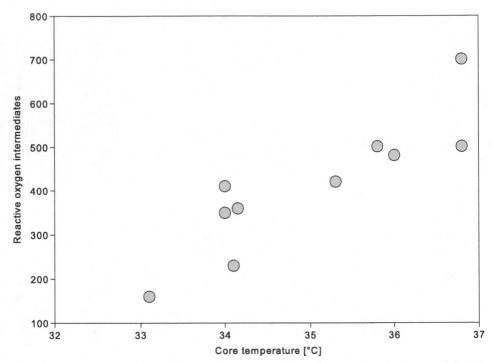

Fig. 18.3 Intraoperative production of reactive oxygen intermediates of neutrophil granulocytes measured in fluorescence units at different core temperatures of patients undergoing colorectal surgery. (Redrawn using data from [197].)

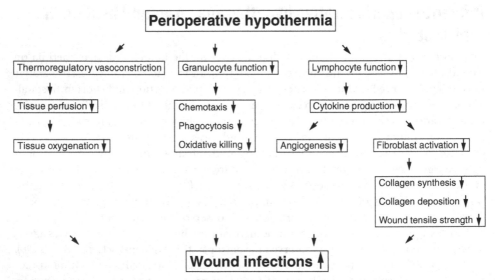

Fig. 18.4 Summary of the pathogenesis of increased wound infection rate caused by perioperative hypothermia.

and collagen deposition near the wound was significantly lower in the routine intraoperative thermal care group. All these results correspond very well with the pathophysiology of wound healing described above.

However, the results of this study were highly debated, especially because a retrospective study in 1999 could not confirm the results [200]. In 2001 a study by Melling et al. [192] was published. In this prospective randomised trial, 421 patients having clean surgery were randomised to either a standard thermal care group without any warming or one of two actively warmed groups (30 minutes of local warming before surgery or 30 minutes of systemic prewarming with a forced-air warming whole-body blanket). A single blinded observer reviewed patients two and six weeks postoperatively and observed the wounds directly. Core temperatures of the patients were normal on the day of admission and increased slightly during local warming 0.13 ± 0.57 °C or systemic prewarming 0.35 ± 0.58 °C. The rate of wound infection was 14% in the group without any warming but only 5% if patients received local or systemic prewarming. Additionally, in the patient group without warming, antibiotics were prescribed in 16% postoperatively, whereas in the prewarmed groups only 7% of the patients were prescribed antibiotics. The results of this study can be explained very well by the effect of local and systemic warming on tissue oxygenation [194].

There has also been another prospective randomised trial studying the effect of local warming on wound healing. In this study on 45 patients after hernia surgery, the ASEPSIS wound score was lower in the warmed groups compared to the control group. However, the results of this study are difficult to judge, because this was only a preliminary study with a small number of patients and the difference in ASEPSIS wound score was caused by one major infection in the control group [201].

Several prospective and retrospective studies have also found an increased risk of wound infection after gastric bypass surgery [202], cholecystectomy [203], trauma laparotomy [204], plastic surgery [205] and wound healing problems [206]. There were also several negative retrospective studies that could not find a significantly increased risk of wound infection due to perioperative hypothermia, for example after abdominal surgery [187, 207], neurosurgery [208], orthopaedic surgery [209], paediatric spinal surgery [210] and caesarean section [211].

However, taking all the information on the pathophysiology and the clinical studies together there is very strong evidence that perioperative hypothermia increases the risk of wound infection [17, 20]. Additionally, perioperative hypothermia is also associated with other infectious complications like pneumonia [187] and sepsis [187, 188].

Chapter

19

Postoperative protein catabolism, length of stay, costs and mortality

Postoperative protein catabolism

Surgery triggers a cascade of events that is usually called the stress response. This stress response is characterised by a release of hormones such as catecholamines and cortisol, and activation of the immune system by cytokines. This leads to insulin resistance and protein catabolism with protein break-down and amino acid oxidation, and a net loss of protein, especially from the skeletal muscles. Patients that develop perioperative hypothermia have increased plasma catecholamine concentrations during and after surgery [179] and as a consequence a higher whole-body protein breakdown and amino acid oxidation with increased urinary nitrogen excretion [212]. This is increased for two to four days postoperatively in patients that develop perioperative hypothermia [213, 214]. The excretion of the amino acid 3-methylhistidine is increased in particular, which is thought to be an indicator of muscle breakdown [214, 215]. Postoperative catabolism and muscle wasting can lead to significant muscle weakness and may delay postoperative mobilisation of the patient.

Perioperative hypothermia increases whole-body and muscle protein breakdown, thus leading to muscle weakness.

Cancer recurrence and establishment of tumour metastasis

Cancer surgery always releases tumour cells into the circulation, and these circulating tumour cells can establish tumour metastasis, depending on the host immune function. Factors that impair immune function during and after the operation may facilitate establishment of tumour metastasis [216]. Perioperative hypothermia induces several changes in immune function [196–198] that impair host defence. In animal experiments, anaesthesia and hypothermia reduce the activity of natural killer cells and lead to a higher retention of tumour cells in the lungs. This leads to more lung metastasis in hypothermic animals [217].

In a follow-up of the milestone study by Kurz *et al.* that studied the effect of hypothermia on wound infection [168], Yücel *et al.* investigated, 5 to 9 years later, if the patients that were assigned to the hypothermia group had more metastasis of their colonic cancer compared to the patients in the normothermia group. They found that cancer-free and overall survival rates were similar in both treatment groups [216].

Mild perioperative hypothermia does not increase recurrent tumours or cancer death.

However, in a large retrospective study in patients with ovarian cancer, perioperative hypothermia was associated with several perioperative complications, such as thromboembolic complications, infections and transfusion. Five-year survival was also reduced [169].

Intensive care unit length of stay

Sometimes hypothermic patients cannot be extubated in the operating room and therefore must be admitted to the intensive care unit. In Germany this is one of the most frequent anaesthesia-related reasons for unplanned admission to intensive care [218]. When patients had to be admitted to the intensive care unit, severe perioperative hypothermia with a core temperature below 34.5 °C was a risk factor for a longer stay in patients undergoing open abdominal aortic aneurysm repair [219]. However, in two other studies, no association between perioperative hypothermia and intensive care unit length of stay could be observed [58, 167].

Length of hospital stay

Perioperative hypothermia has many undesirable effects. Reduced platelet function and impaired plasmatic coagulation increases blood loss and the risk of transfusion [153]. It also increases the risk of pulmonary complications [176] and causes several cardiovascular complications [167, 188]. Additionally, the risk of wound infections [168, 192] and other infectious complications like pneumonia [187] and sepsis [188] is higher. All these factors together may increase the hospital length of stay [140, 168, 188, 219]. Once again, some studies did not observe this effect [58, 139, 161, 167].

Based on the available studies in 2008, NICE in Britain concluded that hypothermia leads to an increase in hospital length of stay [17].

Costs

Several authors have tried to calculate the costs associated with perioperative hypothermia [17]. It is obvious that hypothermia-associated adverse events induce additional costs for the hospital and society. However, different health systems, with their diverse structures, make it extremely difficult to compare prices and costs. The most concise calculation of the costs associated with perioperative hypothermia was performed by NICE using a complex economic model. In brief, the calculation gave the costs shown in Table 19.1 for each adverse consequence of perioperative hypothermia [17]:

In other health care systems with a different economic structure, the costs may be different. However, the costs of wound infections after major surgery or cardiac events are extremely expensive and are of great economic importance.

Table 19.1 Adverse consequences of perioperative hypothermia

Adverse consequences of perioperative hypothermia	Costs (£)
Surgical wound infection after minor surgery	950
Surgical wound infection after major surgery	3858
Transfusion	244
Morbid cardiac event (myocardial ischaemia)	2024
Morbid cardiac event (myocardial infarction)	1674
Morbid cardiac event (cardiac arrest)	2021
Unplanned postoperative mechanical ventilation	1144
Pressure ulcer	1064
PACU length of stay per hour	44
Hospital length of stay per day	275

NICE concluded that perioperative hypothermia induces additional costs to the health system and that the effective prevention of perioperative hypothermia is cost effective, even when the risk of it occurring is low, the risk of cardiac complications is negligible and the anaesthesia duration is short [17].

Mortality

Direct hypothermia-related deaths due to extreme intraoperative hypothermia as happened the 1950s [2] should not occur in operating rooms today. However, even in the 1980s, persistent postoperative hypothermia was associated with mortality. In several studies postoperative hypothermia was associated with a higher mortality [138, 220, 221]. This was sometimes significant in univariate analysis, but not in the subsequent multivariate analysis [139, 219, 222]. In one large retrospective study with more than 45 000 patients, hypothermia was significantly associated with in-hospital mortality [188].

Data are still conflicting, if perioperative hypothermia is independently associated with death. In some large studies there is an association between perioperative hypothermia and mortality.

Chapter

20 Equipment to measure core temperature

Several different technologies are available for measurement of core temperature. These technologies include thermistors, thermocouples, infrared-thermometers and zero-heat-flux thermometers. Mercury-in-glass thermometers, chemical phase-change thermometers and liquid crystal thermometers are not suitable for the measurement of core temperature in the perioperative setting.

Thermistors

Thermistors are widely used to measure core temperature. The technology uses the fact that the electrical resistance of a metal oxide sensor decreases rapidly with an increase in temperature. Newer thermistors use small beads of complex materials [223]. The relatively large changes in electrical resistance make thermistors very sensitive temperature measurement devices [224]. Commonly, the thermistor resistance falls exponentially with increasing temperature (Fig. 20.1).

Therefore, thermistors are connected to an electronic circuit to measure the resistance and to convert the measured resistance into a displayed temperature reading using stored calibration data [223]. With this technology, temperature can be sensed very accurately and the linearity of thermistors is good (Fig. 20.2).

Electronic thermometers – for example for the measurement of oral temperature – sometimes provide a predictive mode that tracks the changing temperature during the measurement process to estimate the final temperature when thermal equilibrium is reached with the surrounding tissue. This predictive mode has the advantage of producing a temperature reading within a few seconds, at the cost of a lower accuracy [223].

Thermocouples

Thermocouples are also widely used to measure core temperature. The technology uses the fact that a small electric potential difference is produced depending on the temperature of the junction of two dissimilar metals. However, the signals from thermocouples are also nonlinear and have to be linearised by calibrated compensating units [34]. Thermocouples are an accurate method for the measurement of temperature (Fig. 20.3).

Infrared-thermometers

Infrared-thermometers are widely used to measure core temperature in patients that are awake. For that purpose special optical sensors have been developed, that are capable of

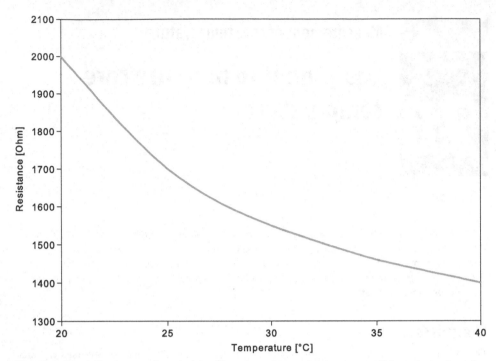

Fig. 20.1 Electrical resistance of a typical thermistor depending on the temperature. (Schematic drawing using data from [224].)

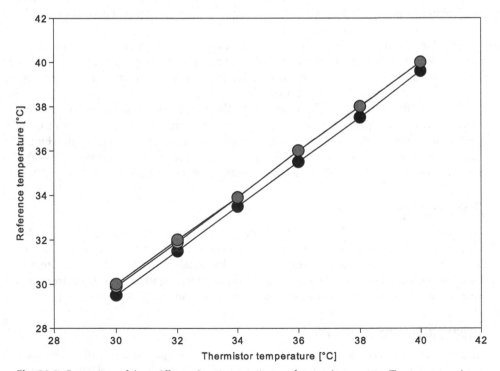

Fig. 20.2 Comparison of three different thermistors against a reference thermometer. The accuracy and linearity of thermistors are very good.

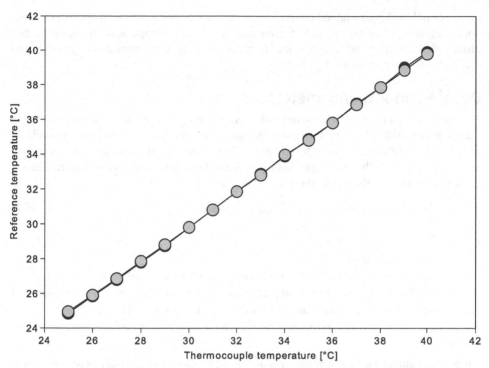

Fig. 20.3 Comparison of two different thermocouples against a reference thermometer. The accuracy of thermocouples is very good.

measuring a portion of the infrared emissions from surfaces within the field of view [223]. The sensor does not have to be in contact with the measured object. The received infrared energy must then be converted into a temperature reading [223]. The calibration of infrared-thermometers is performed by the use of black-body radiators. In general, the technology can measure temperature accurately [33]. However, when the devices are used to measure core temperature at the tympanic membrane, they do not measure only the tympanic temperature, but also that of adjacent parts of the aural canal [33, 223], which are up to 1 °C cooler [223]. Therefore the measured values are adjusted using confidential algorithms from the manufacturer [223].

Zero-heat-flux thermometers

A newer method of measuring core temperature is the use of zero-heat-flux thermometers, which were invented more than 40 years ago. Zero-heat-flux thermometers estimate core temperature from the surface of the lateral forehead of the patient [225]. Under normal conditions, the temperature of the skin depends greatly on ambient conditions. The technique combines a servo-controlled heater with a heat flux transducer that measures the heat flux from the skin to the environment. When the zero-heat-flux thermometer is switched on, the heater warms the skin until the measured heat flux is zero. At this point the skin temperature and the temperature of the tissues below the heat flux transducer are equal [33]. Thereby the zero-heat-flux thermometer creates a small isothermal zone of tissue in which almost no heat transfer to the environment occurs. To minimise the influence of blood-borne lateral convection of heat, the device must be an appropriate size. Following an equilibration period of a few minutes the core temperature is measured and displayed. At the moment zero-heat-flux thermometers are being evaluated extensively and the first results are promising [225–227].

Double-sensor thermometers

Another new method of measuring core temperature is the use of a double-sensor thermometer [228, 229]. The method uses a heat flux transducer placed on the forehead of the patient to estimate core temperature. This heat flux transducer consists of two temperature probes that are separated by an insulator with a known thermal resistance. Core temperature is then essentially calculated as follows [229]:

$$T_{Core} = T_{Skin} + (K_{Sensor}K_{Human\ tissue}^{-1})(T_{Skin} - T_{Sensor}) \qquad (20.1)$$

where
T_{Core} = core temperature [°C]
T_{Skin} = skin temperature under the insulator of the double-sensor [°C]
T_{Sensor} = surface temperature of the double-sensor above the insulator of the sensor [°C]
K_{Sensor} = heat exchange coefficient of the insulator in the sensor [W m^{-2} °C^{-1}]
$K_{Human\ tissue}$ = empirically estimated heat exchange coefficient of the human tissue [W m^{-2} °C^{-1}]

Currently, double-sensor thermometers are being evaluated extensively, with promising results [228, 229].

Chapter

21

Measurement of core temperature

The core temperature of the body is an important vital sign and is an indicator for active metabolism and functioning thermoregulation. Therefore the measurement of the core temperature is an important part of perioperative physiologic monitoring [230]. It is essential to detect perioperative hypothermia, to control the effectiveness of warming therapy [230], to prevent overheating and facilitate detection of malignant hyperthermia [33]. Although core temperature does not completely characterise body heat content and distribution, it is the best single indicator of thermal status in humans [33].

The use of temperature monitoring is a protective factor against hypothermia [58, 59]. Therefore perioperative core temperature monitoring is recommended [17, 19, 20] in patients undergoing general anaesthesia for more than 30 minutes and in all patients whose surgery lasts longer than 1 hour [33].

Definition of the thermal core of the body

The thermal core of the body can be defined as those inner tissues of the body whose temperatures are not changed in their relationship to each other by circulatory adjustments nor by changes in heat dissipation to the environment [31].

This is the actual definition by the Commission for Thermal Physiology of the International Union of Physiological Sciences. Although this is the best available definition of the thermal core of the body, it is not very concrete, especially in the perioperative setting. Under normal conditions, the temperatures of the intra-abdominal organs are not changed in their relationship to each other by circulatory adjustments. Therefore they belong to the thermal core of the body. During abdominal surgery these organs are exposed to the environment and start to dissipate heat to the environment and cool down. In that situation the intra-abdominal organs are no longer part of the thermal core.

It is very important to measure core temperature far away from the surgical site to avoid erroneous measurements.

An ideal system to measure core temperature at a specific site should be small, easy to use, comfortable, fast, continuous, accurate, precise, non-invasive, low energy-consuming and affordable [230]. To date no system and no measurement site fulfils all these criteria.

Measurement sites

The best measurement sites should measure temperature in highly perfused tissues whose temperature is uniform and high compared with the rest of the body [33]. Therefore, temperature is measured in the pulmonary artery or the iliac artery, in the distal oesophagus, directly at the tympanic membrane or in the nasopharynx [230]. These temperature-monitoring sites usually remain very reliable, even during rapid changes in core temperature [33]. However, these measurement sites often cannot be used in conscious patients and even in anaesthetised patients sometimes give erroneous measurements.

Gold standards of core temperature measurement

Pulmonary artery temperature

The pulmonary artery is an extremely well-perfused tissue deep in the trunk of the body and the temperature measured with a thermistor at the tip of the catheter is thought to represent the temperature of the well-perfused tissues of the body.

Advantages
- One of the gold standards for core temperature measurements [33, 230].
- The probe has minimal risk of dislocation.

Potential problems
- Measurement of the pulmonary artery temperature is only possible when a pulmonary artery catheter is used, for example in some patients during cardiac surgery and in some other extremely carefully selected patients.
- Rapid infusion of cold or insufficiently warmed infusions can lead to a rapid drop in blood temperature in the pulmonary artery, which is then not representative of the temperature of the tissues.
- Exposure of intrathoracic organs to the environment, for example during lung surgery, may lead to erroneously low readings [177].

Measurement of the temperature in the pulmonary artery is one of the gold standards of core temperature measurement. However, it is only occasionally available and therefore does not play an important role in clinical core temperature measurement.

Iliac artery temperature

In many countries the pulmonary artery catheter for invasive haemodynamic monitoring has been widely replaced by the transpulmonary thermodilution technique, because the latter is less invasive and provides, in addition to cardiac output measurements, more reliable indicators of preload and the measurement of extravascular lung fluid. The blood temperature in the iliac artery can be measured using a thermistor-tipped arterial catheter that is usually placed in the femoral artery.

Advantages

- The iliac artery is also an extremely well-perfused tissue deep in the trunk of the body and the temperature measured at the tip of the catheter is also thought to represent the temperature of the well-perfused tissues of the body. Under many circumstances the temperature of the iliac artery is identical to the temperature of the pulmonary artery. It is also one of the gold standards for core temperature measurement.
- The probe has only a minimal risk of dislocation.

Potential problems

- Measurement of the iliac artery temperature requires the use of a special thermistor-tipped arterial catheter, which is normally only used in some critically ill patients.
- Rapid infusion of cold or insufficiently warmed infusions can lead to a rapid drop in blood temperature in the iliac artery, which is then not representative of the temperature of the tissues.
- Exposure of pelvic organs to the environment, for example during lower abdominal, gynaecological or urological surgery may lead to erroneously low readings.

> Measurement of the temperature in the iliac artery is also one of the gold standards of core temperature measurement. However, it is only occasionally available and therefore does not play an important role in clinical core temperature measurement.

Oesophageal temperature

Temperature measurement in the distal oesophagus can be measured with a simple probe, an oesophageal stethoscope or a gastric tube with an incorporated temperature sensor. The distal oesophagus is also located deep in the trunk of the body. It is not extremely well perfused, but it is located directly between the left atrium of the heart and the aorta descendens and therefore is only a few millimetres away from the blood in the left atrium and the aorta (Fig. 21.1).

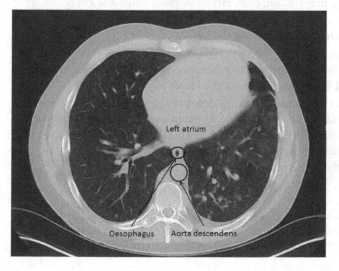

Fig. 21.1 Relationship of the distal oesophagus and the left atrium of the heart and the aorta descendens.

Advantages

Oesophageal temperature is one of the gold standards of core temperature measurement [33, 230].

Positioning of the probe

To get valid measurement results the probe has to be positioned in the distal oesophagus behind the left atrium. This position can be achieved by placing the tip of the probe, during laryngoscopy, 24 to 28 cm below the corniculate cartilages [231] or 36 to 41 cm below the nostril, in adults without laryngoscopy. This distance can be exactly calculated by the formula of Mekjavic and Rempel [232]:

$$\text{Distance from the nostril [cm]} = 0.228 \text{ length [cm]} \tag{21.1}$$

In children, the distance from the corniculate cartilages to the distal oesophagus can be calculated by the following formula [233]:

$$\text{Distance [cm]} = 10 + \frac{2 \times \text{ age [years]}}{3} \tag{21.2}$$

Another way of positioning the oesophageal probe in the distal oesophagus is the use of an oesophageal stethoscope. As the oesophageal stethoscope is progressively inserted, the breath sounds are loudest with no audible heart sounds, then the breath sounds decrease with increasing heart sounds and finally strong heart sounds with weak breath sounds can be heard. The ideal position is 12–16 cm deeper than the position where the best combination of breath and heart sounds can be obtained at the point where the loudest heart sounds can be heard [40]. Positioning the temperature probe behind the heart is essential, because large temperature gradients up to 6 °C can exist in the oesophagus. In the upper or middle oesophagus the temperature is lowered by the influence of the relatively cold air in the trachea [177, 231, 233]. This effect is reduced with the use of heat and moisture exchangers or low-flow and minimal-flow anaesthesia.

Potential problems

- Impossible to use during many nasal, oral, laryngeal procedures and every oesophageal procedure.
- Incorrect low temperature readings during thoracic surgery [177].
- Can be influenced by operations in the upper abdomen.
- Continuous gastric suctioning during abdominal surgery can produce an artefactual lowering of oesophageal temperature measurements of more than 1 °C.
- Can be influenced by oral secretions tracking down to the connection between the probe and the monitor cable. This is possible in the prone position or the sitting position. Thereby the electrical resistance of the temperature measurement system is lowered and an erroneously high temperature (up to 4.8 °C) is displayed.
- Can be placed incorrectly in the trachea, giving false low readings.

To get valid measurement results, the oesophageal temperature probe has to be positioned in the distal oesophagus behind the left atrium. The easiest way to achieve this position is to place the probe 36 to 41 cm below the nostril in the oesophagus in adults.

Tympanic membrane temperature measured with contact thermometry

Tympanic membrane temperature can be measured with soft and pliable temperature probes. The tympanic membrane is located a few centimetres within the scull near the internal carotid artery, which also supplies blood to the hypothalamus. It is only separated from the internal carotid artery by about 1 cm, by the middle ear and an extremely thin bony shell.

Advantages

- Temperature measurement directly at the tympanic membrane is also one of the gold standards of core temperature measurement [33, 230].
- In contrast to many other gold standards, the tympanic membrane temperature is tolerated in conscious patients.

Positioning of the probe

To get valid measurement results, the probe has to be positioned directly on the tympanic membrane. The insertion of a tympanic temperature probe is somewhat more difficult than it sounds [33], because the aural canal is several centimetres long and has a sigmoid form that becomes more tortuous and narrowed in later life. The canal travels first anteriorly, then posteriorly, and finally anteriorly again [234]; additionally, it also travels upwards and downwards (Fig. 21.2). To straighten the cartilaginous part of the external ear canal the ear can be gently pulled upwards and posterior, which makes positioning of the probe easier. Sometimes a bend in the canal is mistaken for the tympanic membrane and the probe is not positioned on the membrane itself [33]. To assure proper positioning the patient should be conscious and a gentle rubbing of the attached wire should be heard as a scratching sound [235]. After the probe is properly positioned, the aural canal should be occluded with cotton and protected externally.

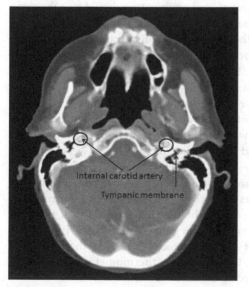

Fig. 21.2 Anatomy of the aural canal and the relationship between the internal carotid artery and the tympanic membrane.

Potential problems

- Cannot be used during some operative procedures on the head.
- It can be difficult to place the probe correctly [33].
- Sometimes the probe is not positioned on the membrane itself.
- Dislocation of the probe during the procedure is possible and cannot be detected easily.
- Earwax or dried blood in the auditory canal can lead to slow responses.
- Earwax can be pushed onto the tympanic membrane by the temperature probe [33].
- It can be influenced by the temperature of the surrounding skin [236]. This can lead to significant errors if the skin of the head is heated by operating lamps, for example during neurosurgery [236].
- It can be influenced by the position of the body and the head. In the lateral position the temperature on the lower side increases whereas that of the upper side decreases.
- Tympanic membrane temperature readings can decrease erroneously after operative exposure of the mastoid bone and cerebellopontine angle [236].
- Perforation of the tympanic membrane is possible [237]. Therefore clinicians sometimes do not place the probe deep enough, so that it does not measure the temperature on the tympanic membrane.

> Although the measurement of core temperature on the tympanic membrane is one of the gold standards of core temperature measurement, this measurement site is not very well suited for clinical practice because correct placement of the probe is cumbersome and there is a risk of injuring the tympanic membrane if repositioning of the patient or the head is needed intraoperatively.

Comparison of different sites of core temperature measurement

In theory, the gold standard measurement sites of core temperature should give the same results and should be interchangeable. When temperature measurements at different sites are compared, most of the time the method developed by Bland and Altman is used. The Bland–Altman plot is a scatterplot of the difference between the two measurements against the mean of the two measurements (Fig. 21.3).

When both sites give the same results, the bias and the limits of agreement should be zero. However, this is only true in theory and no study has ever shown this. For example, in intensive care patients without any interference of the measurement by surgery, the mean bias between pulmonary artery temperature and oesophageal temperature was 0.1 °C and the limits of agreement were ±0.6 °C [238]. It can be concluded that in reality there is some unavoidable scattering of the data, even when so-called gold standard measurement sites are compared. This scattering comes from measurement errors by incorrect placement of the probes or temporary thermal imbalances in the core of the body. This must be kept in mind when other measurement sites are compared with the gold standard sites. It has been proposed that a clinically acceptable level of accuracy could be that the combined inaccuracy (bias and single standard deviation) of a site–thermometer combination should not exceed 0.5 °C [33]. This is hard to achieve.

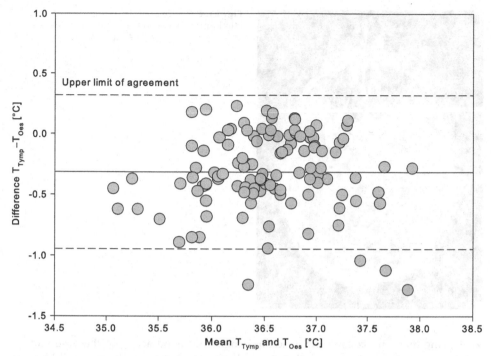

Fig. 21.3 Bland–Altman plot of a comparison of the tympanic and oesophageal temperature. The comparison shows the mean bias (solid line) and upper and lower limits of agreement (± 2 standard deviations). In this comparison the tympanic membrane temperature was 0.3 °C lower than the oesophageal temperature (mean bias -0.3 °C) and the limits of agreement were ±0.6 °C.

Other sites for core temperature measurement

All gold-standard sites for core temperature measurement have several drawbacks in clinical practice. Pulmonary artery temperature or iliac artery temperature are rarely available, tympanic membrane temperature measured with contact thermometry is cumbersome and oesophageal temperature is not sensible during thoracic and upper abdominal surgery. Therefore in Europe core temperature is monitored <1% in the pulmonary artery and only in about 10% in the oesophagus [239]. In a survey in Germany, the use of all gold standard measurement sites together was below 5% [240]. To overcome this problem, core temperature can be estimated with reasonable accuracy using other measurement sites.

Nasopharyngeal temperature

Temperature is measured at the nasopharyngeal mucosa deep within the skull only about 9 to 13 mm away from the internal carotid artery, which also supplies blood to the hypothalamus (Fig. 21.4) [241].

Advantages

- Nasopharyngeal temperature shows a good correlation to the pulmonary artery temperature [242], tympanic temperature and oesophageal temperature [243], as well as a clinically acceptable level of accuracy [242, 243]. Therefore some authors judge it to be as good as the gold standard measurement sites [33].

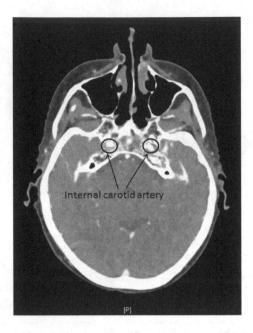

Fig. 21.4 Anatomy of the nasopharynx and relationship between the internal carotid artery and the nasopharyngeal mucosa.

- During many procedures the anaesthesiologist has good access to the head and to the nasopharyngeal probe, so that the probe can easily be repositioned if dislocation occurs.
- Additionally, it is possible to measure nasopharyngeal temperature with a magnetic resonance imaging (MRI)-compatible temperature probe, for example during diagnostic MRI or during neurosurgical procedures in open MRI.

Positioning of the probe

Nasopharyngeal temperature probes should be inserted 9 to 20 cm past the nares through the inferior meatus to obtain core temperature [241, 244]. The probe and a cover should be fixated with tape to avoid dislocation.

Potential problems

- Cannot be used during some operative procedures on the head.
- Is often not placed optimally. In a study by Lee *et al.* [241], only about 40% of all nasopharyngeal probes were placed optimally. Some probes were placed in the nasal cavity, while others were even placed in the hypopharynx, which led to slightly lower temperature readings. Some covers for temperature probes have a length of only 8 cm, which hinders optimal placement at 9–10 cm depth. Additionally, nasopharyngeal probes normally have no length markers to enable correct insertion of the probe [241].
- Can be influenced by air in patients who are breathing through their nostrils [33, 177].
- Can give wrong readings if dislocated. Dislocation can occur with the probe moving out or moving too deep, for example together with a boogie or a gastric tube.
- If a cover is used there is a potential risk of aspiration of the cover if it is not adequately secured.

- Inserting a probe into the nasopharynx can cause epistaxis [177, 241] in about 2.7%. In some rare cases excessive bleeding has occurred. It is important to insert the probe gently without any force, but it is also important to get contact with the mucosa. If this is not possible it is wise to swap nostrils.

Nasopharyngeal temperature is useful during many procedures and can be easily obtained. In clinical practice it is acceptably accurate. Therefore, it is the most used site for temperature monitoring in Germany [240] and Europe [239].

Oral or sublingual temperature

Oral, or more precisely sublingual, temperature measures core temperature in the posterior sublingual pocket. This region is very well vascularised and if the probe is located correctly under the tongue it is shielded from the surrounding air.

Advantages

- Sublingual temperature measurement of core temperature is applicable and adequately accurate in awake and cooperative patients, but also in patients under general anaesthesia. [245].
- It has the advantage that it is very well tolerated in conscious patients and therefore can be used throughout the whole perioperative period [245].
- It is only minimally invasive.

Positioning of the probe

It is important to position the temperature probe under the tongue in the posterior sublingual pocket. It is not adequate to position the probe somewhere in the mouth, because the temperature reading will be erroneously low if the probe is located in the air.

Potential problems

- Cannot be used during some operative procedures on the head.
- The probe is often not placed optimally and fixation of the probe under the tongue during anaesthesia is difficult, impractical or even impossible [177]. It is also difficult or impossible to get a reliable temperature reading in uncooperative awake patients.
- If a cover is used there is a potential risk of aspiration of the cover if it is not adequately secured.

Sublingual temperature can be measured in the posterior sublingual pocket. It has a clinically acceptable accuracy.

Zero-heat-flux or double-sensor thermometer temperature measurement at the forehead

These thermometers measure core temperature from the skin of the forehead.

Advantages

- The device offers the opportunity to measure core temperature non-invasively throughout the whole perioperative period without changing the measurement site.
- At the moment these thermometers are still under evaluation, but the initial results are promising and it seems that they are or will be an accurate method for the measurement of temperature [225–229].
- The risk of dislocation is small.

Positioning of the probe

The probe just has to be applied to the lateral forehead.

Potential problems

- Cannot be used during some operative procedures on the head.
- The accuracy of these new technologies has not been established in many different clinical situations yet.
- Expensive at the moment.

> Zero-heat-flux or double-sensor thermometer temperature measurements are a new promising technology, but the accuracy of this technology has not yet been established in many different clinical situations.

Bladder temperature

Bladder temperature is measured in the bladder with the use of an indwelling Foley catheter a few centimetres inside the trunk of the body.

Advantages

- The probe is fixated very well and the risk of dislocation is minimal.
- The measurement of bladder temperature is very convenient in the postoperative phase in the PACU or ICU and is often used as a measure of core temperature in Germany [240].
- Bladder temperature is an accurate measure of core temperature in the postoperative phase [246] and the ICU. Comparisons with the pulmonary artery temperature revealed a low bias with a low single standard deviation [238, 247].

Positioning of the probe

The probe is incorporated in the Foley catheter and no special positioning is required.

Potential problems

- Measurement of the bladder temperature requires the use of a special thermistor-tipped Foley catheter. The insertion of a Foley catheter is an invasive procedure and only sensible when the indication for a Foley catheter is given.
- After placement of the probe, several minutes are needed to get reliable results because after insertion of the catheter, the balloon at the tip of catheter is filled with 10 ml of

cold fluid. Only after equilibration of this fluid with the surrounding body temperature are the measurement results reliable.

- Measuring bladder temperature is not sensible during urogenital or lower abdominal surgery [177, 248].
- During surgery, the accuracy of bladder temperature sometimes depends on urinary flow [248, 249], with low urinary flows decreasing the accuracy of readings.

Bladder temperature is useful during many procedures and very convenient in the postoperative phase. In clinical practice it is acceptably accurate, except during urogenital or lower abdominal surgery. Therefore, it is the one of most used sites for temperature monitoring [240].

Rectal temperature

Rectal temperature is measured a few centimetres inside the trunk of the body.

Advantages

- Rectal temperature is a fairly accurate measure of core temperature in the postoperative phase [246] and the ICU. Comparisons with the pulmonary artery temperature revealed a low bias with an acceptable single standard deviation [238]. In children, rectal temperature does not differ from oesophageal temperature [250].

Positioning of the probe

The probe just has to be positioned at least 8 cm deep in the rectum. The probe and a disposable cover should be taped to the patient's buttocks to prevent displacement and the position of the probe should be checked after positioning.

Potential problems

- Temperature in the rectum is often described as being 0.2 to 0.6 °C higher than other core measurement sites.
- Rectal temperature can be influenced by heat-producing flora in the rectum, faeces or cold blood returning from the legs.
- Even if reusable probes are used with a cover they have a high risk of contamination.
- Potential small risk of perforation of the rectum.
- Less accurate than bladder temperature, especially during rapid changes in core temperature [33, 246]
- The probe cannot be fixated very well and the risk of dislocation is high, especially after positioning or repositioning of the patient. If dislocation occurs it is nearly impossible to correct the position of the probe because there is no access to it.
- In the PACU the probe is prone to come out when the patient wakes and starts to move, and the probe is uncomfortable for the conscious patient.
- Not suitable during urogenital and lower abdominal surgery [177].

Rectal temperature is less accurate than bladder temperature and has a high risk of dislocation.

Tympanic membrane temperature measured with infrared thermometry

Tympanic membrane temperature measured with infrared thermometry measures a portion of the infrared emissions from the tympanic membrane and adjacent parts of the aural canal within the field of view and converts this into a temperature reading [223]. Because the aural canal is up to 1 °C cooler than the tympanic membrane, the measured values are adjusted by confidential algorithms from the manufacturer [223].

Advantages

- Temperature measurement with infrared thermometry is fast, convenient and non-invasive.

Positioning of the probe

To get the best possible measurement results, the device has to be directed towards the tympanic membrane. This can be difficult or even impossible because the aural canal has a sigmoid form that becomes more tortuous and narrowed in later life [234]. It is best to straighten the cartilaginous part of the external ear by pulling the ear upwards and posterior.

Potential problems

- Tympanic membrane temperature measurement with infrared thermometry measures a large portion of the aural canal (Fig. 21.5) and therefore is inaccurate in most studies [33, 251]. However, some studies have shown acceptable accuracy.
- The accuracy depends on ear canal morphology and visibility of the tympanic membrane.
- The accuracy of tympanic membrane temperature measurement with infrared thermometry depends very much on the handling of the device. The following handling problems are associated with lower accuracy:
  - Repeated measurements over short time intervals [251, 252].
  - Positioning of the device in the auditory canal before taking the temperature [251, 252]

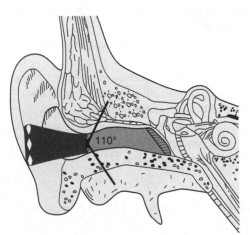

Fig. 21.5 The aural canal with the positioned infrared thermometer. The grey area shows the area from which infrared emissions are detected. This is mainly the auditory canal and not the tympanic membrane. (Reproduced from *Fritz U, Rohrberg M, Lange C, Weyland W, Bräuer A, Braun U.* Infrarot-Temperaturmessung in Gehörgang mit dem DIATEK 9000 Instatemp und dem DIATEK 9000 Thermoguide. Einflussgrössen und Vergleich mit anderen Methoden der Temperaturmessung des Körperkerns. Anaesthesist 1996; **45**: 1059–1066 with permission of Springer [251].)

- Rotation of the device out of the standard position [251, 252]
- Lack of experience with the device [252].

- Some degree of earwax does not reduce the accuracy of the device [252], whereas complete obstruction of the auditory canal by earwax lowers the temperature reading about 0.5 °C.
- Major ear surgery, such as canal wall down surgery, has a significant influence on the result of tympanic membrane temperature measured with infrared thermometry.
- Can only be used for spot checks and not for continuous temperature monitoring.

Tympanic membrane temperature measured with infrared thermometry is too inaccurate for perioperative use.

Temporal artery temperature

Temporal artery temperature was developed to measure the blood temperature of the superficial temporal artery through the skin by infrared radiation measurement. It records the highest skin temperature of the forehead and temporal region and calculates core temperature by the use of a proprietary algorithm that compensates for ambient temperature [253].

Advantages
- Temperature measurement with a temporal artery thermometer is fast and non-invasive.

Positioning of the probe
It is recommended to position the thermometer on the centre of the patient's forehead and then slide it across the forehead to the lateral hairline and the region behind the earlobe [253].

Potential problems
- The devices are too inaccurate for perioperative use [33, 253].
- Can only be used for spot checks and not for continuous temperature monitoring.

Temporal artery temperature measurements are too inaccurate for perioperative use.

Skin surface and axillary temperature

Skin-surface temperatures are significantly lower than core temperature and are dependent on the balance of heat transport to the skin and heat loss to the environment. Therefore skin surface temperature is not a good measure of core temperature [33]. Axillary temperature has a low accuracy in the postoperative phase and is also not a good measure of core temperature. It can be a reasonable substitute for oral temperature in patients in whom oral temperature measurement is unsuitable.

Skin surface temperature and axillary temperature have a low accuracy and are not good measures of core temperature.

Forced-air warmers

22

> Forced-air warmers are also called convective air warmers. The devices are a very well-accepted method for preventing hypothermia in surgical patients because of their documented efficacy, low cost and ease of use [254].

History

The first construction and clinical application of a forced-air warmer was published in 1973 by Lewis [4]. However, it took until 1988 for the first commercially available forced-air warmers to be introduced into clinical practice.

Efficacy

Forced-air warming is a very useful method of preventing perioperative hypothermia. Numerous studies prove the efficacy of forced-air warmers during many surgical procedures and only a small number of these studies are cited here [54, 163, 166, 168, 170, 255]. Therefore forced-air warming is the most frequently used warming device in Germany [240] and Europe [239].

Technology of forced-air warmers

Forced-air warmers consist of a power unit – also called controller – and a blanket that delivers warm air to the patient's body surface that is covered by it. The power unit normally incorporates a microbial air filter, an electric heater, motor and fan to generate an air flow that is delivered via a hose downstream to a compatible inflatable blanket. The heating temperature of the power unit can normally be selected to several preset temperatures. Older power units control this temperature setting by one or two thermostats at the exit of the power unit, whereas newer power units control the air temperature directly at the end of the nozzle, a more satisfying and safer arrangement. If too high a temperature is detected by the thermostats, the power units visually and/or audibly alarm and shut down automatically.

For preoperative warming, forced-air warmers are most often used in combination with full-body blankets [256, 257], upper-body blankets positioned lengthwise over the whole body of the patient [102] or warming gowns [258, 259], whereas intraoperatively, upper-body blankets are commonly preferred [260]. For postoperative rewarming, forced-air warmers are most often used in combination with full-body blankets [50, 261]. However, in recent years, several other types of blanket have been developed especially for intraoperative use to enable the largest possible surface area to be warmed during surgery. At the moment the following types of blankets exist:

- Upper-body blankets covering the chest and the arms
- Extra-large upper-body blankets for obese patients
- Poncho blankets covering the back, the chest and the arms
- Lower-body blankets covering both legs and the lower abdomen
- Torso blankets covering only the chest and the abdomen
- Several underbody blankets that are used underneath the patient
- Surgical access blankets, which are full-body blankets with an area removed in the centre to allow surgical access
- Chest access blankets
- Cath lab blankets
- Sterile cardiac access blankets
- Several paediatric underbody blankets
- Some other rarely used types.

The blankets can be single-use or reusable blankets. Materials used are plastic, polypropylene, polypropylene/polyethylene or fabric. On the patient contact side the blankets are permeable to air. This is achieved either through holes or slits, or by air-permeable blanket fabric [260].

Physical background of forced-air warmers

It makes sense to understand the basic physical background of warming devices to be able to select the best option for the patient. To study this requires constant and reproducible experimental conditions and the ability to vary single factors systematically. Such control is not feasible in patients or volunteers, but it is possible in manikins [262] that have been developed to measure heat exchange and validated against human volunteers [263]. The results of manikin evaluations of forced-air warmers show very reliable results, comparable to those in human volunteers [262, 264]. Therefore the physical background of these devices will be shown based on manikin evaluations.

The power unit

Heat flow produced by the power units can be calculated as:

$$\dot{Q} = F\Delta T c \rho \tag{22.1}$$

where
$\dot{Q}$ = heat flow [W]
F = air flow [l s^{-1}]
ΔT = temperature gradient between the nozzle and the room [°C]
c = specific heat capacity of air [J g^{-1} °C^{-1}]
ρ = air density at the nozzle temperature [g l^{-1}].

This equation shows that the heat flow produced by the power unit depends entirely on the air temperature at the nozzle and the air flow. The specific heat capacity of air and the

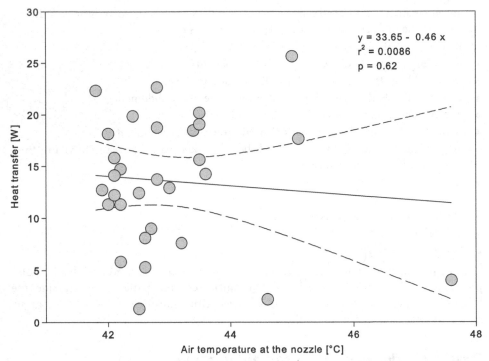

Fig. 22.1 Influence of the nozzle temperature of the power unit on the heat transfer of forced-air warmer upper-body blankets to the surface of a manikin. Data from two manikin investigations with regression line and 95% confidence intervals [254, 262] of 30 combinations of power units and upper-body blankets.

air density are physical constants. Compared to water, the specific heat capacity of air is about four times lower. This is one of the major drawbacks of forced-air warmers because a low specific heat capacity leads to low heat transfer. Increasing air temperature using the power unit increases the heat flow to the blanket. The maximum air temperatures at the nozzle range between 41.5 and 47.6 °C in power units [254, 261, 262, 265]. Due to current restrictions by international standards the temperature is now limited to 43 °C. The air flow of the power units ranges between 7.4 and 26.2 l s^{-1} [254, 261, 265]. The different air flows of the power units result in heat flows to the blankets of between 180 and 623 W [254, 261, 262, 265].

It could be expected that power units producing a higher air temperature at the nozzle would create a higher heat flow to the blanket and therefore would increase heat transfer to the body surface. This effect was seen to a very slight degree in a manikin study with full-body blankets [261]; however, in two manikin studies with upper-body blankets [254, 262], the maximal air temperature at the nozzle of the power unit did not significantly influence the heat transfer from the blanket to the manikin (Fig. 22.1).

The air flow created by the power units influences heat transfer from full-body blankets to the surface of the body [261], but there is no relationship between the air flow at the nozzle of the power unit and the resulting heat transfer with upper-body blankets [254]. At first sight the differing influences of air temperature and air flow on the heat transfer of full-body blankets and upper-body blankets are puzzling. The difference in size of the upper-body blankets and full-body blankets is probably the reason for the observed variations. In large full-body blankets and presumably in large underbody blankets, a high air flow is essential to distribute the heat from the nozzle to the distant parts of the blanket. The higher the air flow, the better the distribution of the heated air inside the blanket [260]. In contrast, in the much smaller upper-body blankets, and presumably in paediatric blankets, a high air flow does not really help to distribute the heat in the blanket [8]. This may explain why in a clinical study with different forced-air warmers using upper-body blankets no difference was found between two forced-air warmers, although one of the two studied power units had a much higher air flow at the nozzle [266].

The forced-air warmer blanket

The forced-air warmer blanket is connected to the nozzle of the power unit. It distributes the heated air to the covered body surface. The patient contact surface is permeable to air and the heated air exits through the blanket and moves over the patient's skin, thereby transferring heat by convection. Additionally some heat is transferred by conduction and radiation [260]. The physics of this heat exchange process can be described as:

$$\dot{Q} = h \Delta T A \tag{22.2}$$

where
$\dot{Q}$ = heat transfer [W]
h = heat exchange coefficient [W m^{-2} °C^{-1}]
ΔT = mean temperature gradient between the blanket and the body surface [°C]
A = heat exchange area [m^2]

The heat exchange coefficient h defines the efficiency of all the heat exchange mechanisms (radiation, convection and conduction) between the blanket and the body surface. It can be determined in a manikin by measuring the heat flux per unit area with heat flux transducers, and simultaneously measuring the temperature gradient between the blanket and the body surface over a range of temperature differences. The heat exchange coefficient is then calculated by linear regression analysis as the slope of heat exchange per unit area as a function of the blanket–surface temperature gradient (Fig. 22.2) [262].

The mean temperature gradient ΔT is dependent on the surface temperature of the body and the efficacy of the system, and is the driving force for the heat exchange. In patients, the mean skin temperature under a forced-air warming blanket is in the range 36–38 °C [267]. To get the mean temperature gradient, a range of temperature differences can be created experimentally and the resulting temperature differences between the blanket and the surface can be plotted as a function of the temperature of the surface; a regression line is used to calculate their relationship (Fig. 22.3).

Interestingly, there is a large scattering of the data and the data points of the four temperature settings in this experiment show a slightly skewed distribution. This can be explained by the fact that directly at the nozzle the air temperature is high which in turn leads to a high heat transfer and also increases the surface temperature in this area. In contrast, in more distant parts of the blanket the air temperature is lower, because due to

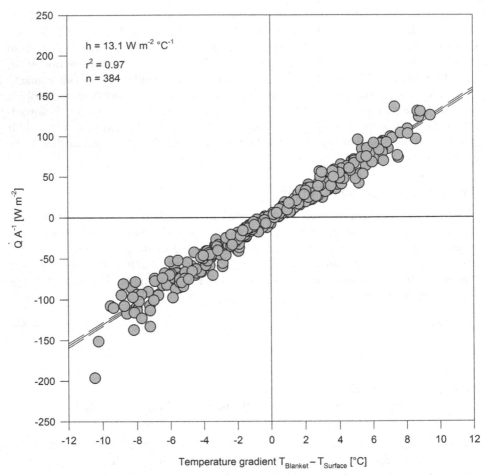

Fig. 22.2 Determination of the heat exchange coefficient of the Warm-Gard® Portable Warmer with a reusable lower-body blanket. The slope of the regression line represents the heat exchange coefficient. (Reproduced from: Bräuer A, English MJ, Lorenz N, Steinmetz N, Perl T, Braun U and Weyland W. Comparison of forced-air warming systems with lower body blankets using a copper manikin of the human body. *Acta Anaesthesiol Scand* 2003; **47**: 58–64 [265] with kind permission of John Wiley & Sons Inc.)

the low specific heat capacity of air the heat is already lost to the surface or to the environment. This leads to a lower temperature gradient and therefore a lower surface temperature. The inhomogeneity of the air temperature in the forced-air warmer blankets can be shown very well in upper-body blankets (Fig. 22.4).

The heat exchange coefficients for different forced-air warmer blankets vary by a factor of three and range between 12.5 $Wm^{-2} \degree C^{-1}$ and 36.2 $Wm^{-2} \degree C^{-1}$ [254, 261, 262, 265]. The temperature gradients between the blanket and surface depend on the surface temperature. The lower the surface temperature, the higher the temperature gradient. It also depends on the type of blanket used. For surface temperatures of 36 to 38 °C, mean temperature gradients of 0.49 to 3.31 °C were observed for upper-body blankets [262]. The mean temperature gradients for lower-body blankets was 0.62 to 2.48 °C [265] and for full-body blankets they ranged between –0.06 and 2.12 °C [261].

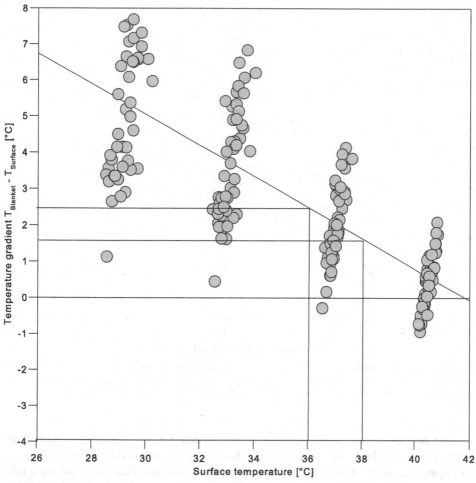

Fig. 22.3 Determination of the mean temperature gradient for surface temperatures of 36 °C and 38 °C for the Warm-Gard® Portable Warmer with a reusable lower-body blanket. (Reproduced from: *Bräuer A, English MJ, Lorenz N, Steinmetz N, Perl T, Braun U and Weyland W*. Comparison of forced-air warming systems with lower body blankets using a copper manikin of the human body. *Acta Anaesthesiol Scand* 2003; **47**: 58–64 [265] with kind permission of John Wiley & Sons Inc.)

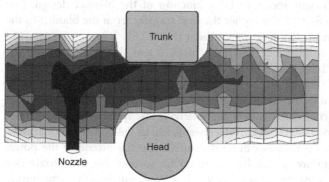

Fig. 22.4 Temperature distribution in an upper-body forced-air warming blanket. The highest temperatures (black) appear near the nozzle on the left side, whereas more distant from the nozzle temperatures are getting lower (dark grey) and lower (light grey). (Redrawn and modified from [268].)

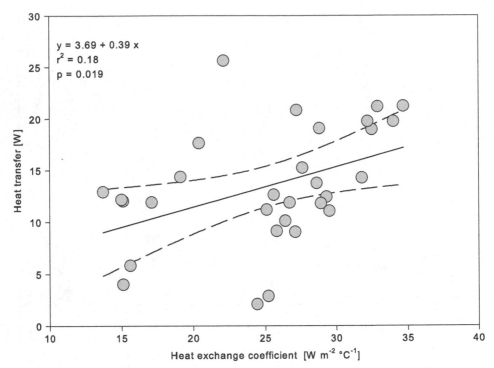

Fig. 22.5 Influence of the heat exchange coefficient on the heat transfer of forced-air warming blankets to the surface of a manikin. Data are from several manikin studies with 30 combinations of upper-body blankets with regression line and 95% confidence intervals. (Redrawn and modified using data from [254, 262].)

The last important parameter that is responsible for heat transfer in forced-air warmers is the body surface area covered. This can be estimated to be about 0.35 m² for an upper-body blanket, 0.54 m² for a lower-body blanket and about 1.21 m² for a full-body blanket.

The equation $\dot{Q} = h\ \Delta T\ A$ shows that there are only three factors that influence the heat transfer of forced-air warmers: the heat exchange coefficient, the mean temperature gradient between the blanket and the body surface, and the body surface area covered by the forced-air warmer blanket.

The heat exchange coefficient seems to be a function of the blanket design. The higher the heat exchange coefficient, the higher the heat transfer from the blanket to the surface will be for a given mean temperature gradient (Fig. 22.5).

The mean temperature gradient between the blanket and the body surface also significantly influences the heat transfer. The higher the mean temperature gradient, the higher the heat transfer (Fig. 22.6).

However, as an additional factor, the homogeneity of temperature distribution within the blanket is of great importance. Because of the relatively low specific heat capacity of air, there is a temperature drop in every blanket as heat is lost to the body surface and the environment. The highest temperatures can be measured near the nozzle of the power unit and the lowest temperature is usually measured far away from the nozzle (see Fig. 22.4). A simple parameter for the homogeneity of heat distribution is the temperature

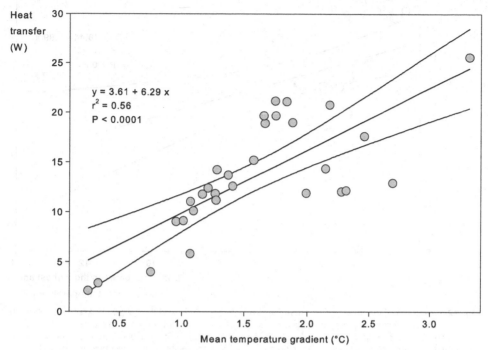

Heat transfer (W)

y = 3.61 + 6.29 x
r² = 0.56
P < 0.0001

Mean temperature gradient (°C)

Fig. 22.6 Influence of the mean temperature gradient on the heat transfer of forced-air warming blankets to the surface of a manikin. Data are from several manikin studies with 30 combinations of upper-body blankets with regression line and 95% confidence intervals. (Reproduced with permission from Wolters Kluwer: Bräuer A and Quintel M. Forced-air warming: technology, physical background and practical aspects. Curr Opin Anaesthesiol 2009; **22**: 769–774 [260].)

difference measured between the highest and the lowest blanket temperature. The lower this temperature difference is, the better the performance of the blanket [254]. Astonishingly, this difference ranges between 2.5 °C and 10 °C [260] in upper-body blankets and between 2.8 °C and 16.9 °C in full-body blankets, indicating that there are relevant differences in blanket design that markedly influence the performance of the blankets (Fig. 22.7).

Normally mean skin temperature of an anesthetised human without forced-air warming is about 32–34 °C. If the air temperature of the power unit is about 43 °C at the nozzle, cooling of the skin occurs when the temperature gradient inside the blanket exceeds 9 °C. Therefore a temperature gradient of more than 9 °C is not acceptable and must be considered as an insufficient design of forced-air warmer blanket.

The area that is covered by the blanket is also of utmost importance. The larger the area, the better the efficacy of the forced-air warming system. The reason for this is that forced-air warmers not only transfer heat to the body, they also reduce the heat losses from the covered body surface area to zero (Fig. 22.8).

The fact that the skin under a forced-air warming blanket is no longer the most important source of heat loss, but a source of heat gain, changes the heat balance of the body considerably. The elimination of the heat losses in the treated area is mainly responsible for the efficacy of forced-air warmers and not the heat transfer to the body. This is the reason for the observed higher efficacy of larger forced-air warming blankets.

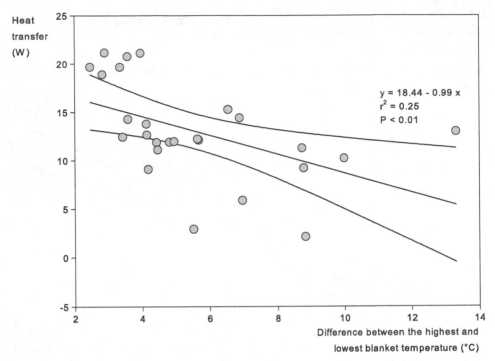

$$y = 18.44 - 0.99\,x$$
$$r^2 = 0.25$$
$$P < 0.01$$

Fig. 22.7 Influence of the temperature difference between the highest and the lowest blanket temperature on the heat transfer of forced-air warming blankets to the surface of a manikin. Data are from several manikin studies with 25 combinations of upper-body blankets with regression line and 95% confidence intervals. (Reproduced with permission from Wolters Kluwer: Bräuer A and Quintel M. Forced-air warming: technology, physical background and practical aspects. Curr Opin Anaesthesiol 2009; **22**: 769–774 [260].)

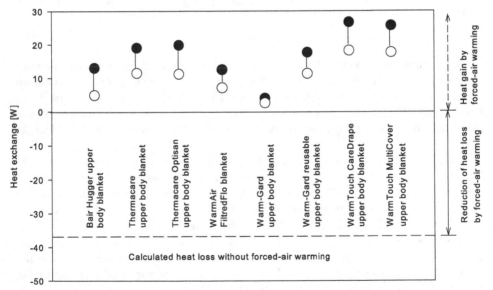

Fig. 22.8 Heat exchange between several forced-air warmer upper-body blankets and a manikin at calculated surface temperatures of 36 °C (black circles) and 38 °C (white circles). The heat gain by the different forced-air warming systems is compared to the calculated heat loss from the body surface at a skin temperature of 32 °C. It can be clearly seen that the reduction in heat loss is more important than the heat gain by the forced-air warmer blanket. (Reproduced from: Bräuer A, English MJM, Steinmetz N, Lorenz N, Perl T, Braun U and Weyland W. Comparison of forced-air warming systems with upper-body blankets using a copper manikin of the human body. *Acta Anaesthesiol Scand* 2002; **46**: 965–972 [262] with kind permission of John Wiley & Sons Inc.)

In general forced-air warmers with upper-body blankets covering about 0.35 m² can transfer about 2.6 to 26.6 W to the body. This results in a change in the heat balance of about 48–72 W [262]. Forced-air warmers with lower-body blankets cover a larger area of about 0.54 m² and can transfer about 8–18.3 W to the body. This results in a larger change in the heat balance of about 78–88.3 W [265]. Full-body blankets covering about 1.21 m² can transfer 8.8 W up to 44.4 W and can lead to a change in the heat balance of 121.9–175.1 W [261].

Practical aspects

The efficacy of a forced-air warmer is mainly determined by the area of the skin that is covered by the blanket, due to the larger effect on the heat balance. Therefore it is important to use the largest blanket that can be applied for the planned operative procedure.

The design of the blanket itself is important for performance. A satisfactory design of forced-air warmer blanket can be detected simply by measuring or feeling the temperature difference between the highest and the lowest blanket temperature.

The temperature difference between the highest and the lowest blanket temperature should be as low as possible to ensure a homogeneous distribution of heat.
    If the power unit of the forced-air warmer is mainly used with large blankets like full-body blankets, surgical access blankets or underbody blankets, it is also important that the power unit has a high air flow to distribute the heated air inside the blanket. If the power unit of the forced-air warmer is mainly used with smaller blankets like upper-body blankets or paediatric blankets then the air flow of the power unit is of minor importance.

Potential problems of forced-air warming

Inadequate warming power in some situations

There is no doubt that forced-air warming is a powerful method for preventing perioperative hypothermia. However, in many of these studies infusion warming or prewarming was also used. There are some studies showing that forced-air warming alone, without infusion warming, can be ineffective [269] and there are also several studies showing that the use of forced-air warming without prewarming of the patient can be ineffective [140, 256, 258]. The main reason for the insufficient efficacy of forced-air warming as the sole measure is the limited influence of small forced-air warmer blankets on the heat balance. Under the relatively normal conditions of an operating room, the heat balance for a minimally dressed person is about –100 to –120 W. This heat balance is changed with a forced-air warmer and an upper-body blanket by about 48–72 W [262] and therefore the heat balance is still negative. With the use of an forced-air warmer with a lower-body blanket the change in the heat balance is about 78–88.3 W [265]. Together with some kind of insulation this can lead to an even heat balance. However, if larger amounts of insufficiently warmed fluids are administered, the heat balance will again be negative.

Therefore, in general it is not enough to use a forced-air warmer intraoperatively. It is important to use it in the right way. Patients should be prewarmed [258] and during the operation the largest blanket that is possible for the operation should be applied [270, 271]. If large amounts of fluids are used during the procedure forced-air warming must be combined with fluid warming because forced-air warming is not powerful enough to compensate for the heat losses occurring by the infusion of large amounts of cold fluids. Supplemental conductive warming over the back can also be helpful.

Overheating

Especially during longer operations [140] or during paediatric operations [104, 272] forced-air warming can lead to undesired overheating of the patients if the temperature of the power unit is not turned down.

As a rule of thumb it is sensible to reduce the temperature of the power unit to 34 °C when the core temperature rises above 37.2 °C.

Risk of burns

Forced-air warming is a remarkably safe procedure if used correctly. There are about 15 to 25 million uses per year and only single cases of burns per year have been reported [260]. The risk of burns is very small and is substantially outweighed by the benefits of forced-air warming. Under normal conditions a skin temperature of less than 43 °C is safe. A skin temperature of more than 43 °C will not be reached if a correct working power unit is used in combination with an adequate blanket [260].

Burns with forced-air warmers have been reported for the following situations:

- Misusing a power unit without an attached blanket and directing the hose under a normal hospital blanket or operating drape [273, 274]. This is called 'free hosing' and is clearly a device misuse. In the American Society of Anesthiologists (ASA) closed claims database, 15 burns resulting from the use of forced-air warmers were documented from 1995 to 2010. In 13 of the 15 cases the power unit was used without an attached blanket and the most common location of burns were the buttocks and lower extremities [275]. Severe third-degree burns have been observed when 'free-hosing' was performed (Fig. 22.9) [273] and in one case ended in an above-knee amputation.
- Direct contact of the nozzle with the skin [274]. This can cause burns because the nozzle is one of the warmest parts of the device and the heat exchanging mechanism with the skin is conduction, which is more efficient than convection [49, 52, 276]. Additionally, pressure can be applied to the nozzle, therefore further increasing the risk of burns, because the combination of heat and pressure lowers the threshold for burn injuries significantly [260].
- Forced-air warming of ischaemic limbs (for example during cross clamping of the artery) or during poor circulation. A child undergoing cardiac catheterisation experienced a third-degree burn of the leg probably due to reduced perfusion of the leg by sheaths placed in the groin vessels and low cardiac output [277]. In another case a child experienced burns during correction of transposition of the great arteries with the

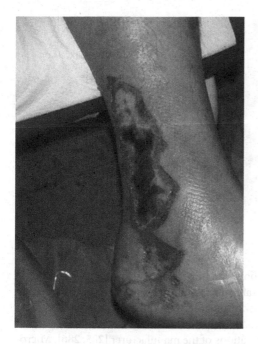

Fig. 22.9 Third-degree burn injury on a patient's left ankle after he was warmed with a forced-air warmer without an attached blanket for two hours after coronary artery bypass surgery. (Reproduced from Uzun G, Mutluoglu M, Evinc R, Ozdemir Y, Sen H. Severe burn injury associated with misuse of forced-air warming device. J Anesth 2010; **24**: 980–981 with permission of Springer [273].)

use of cardiopulmonary bypass. However, it is important to mention that even in this patient population forced-air warming is usually safe [278].

- Obstructed air flow inside the blanket [279].
- Use with the wrong blanket [274].
- Use in small children [274].
- However, there are also some case reports of minor burns with forced-air warmers where the devices were used correctly [280, 281].

Pressure ulcer

There has been a case report of an intraoperative full-thickness pressure ulcer in a patient undergoing transapical aortic valve implantation with an underbody forced-air warming blanket [282]. The procedure was complicated by severe hypotension and bradycardia, so that cardiopulmonary resuscitation had to be initiated and after several minutes of cardiopulmonary resuscitation an emergency median sternotomy was performed to allow cardiopulmonary bypass. After successful resuscitation, the patient recovered for a few days, but experienced a full-thickness pressure ulcer of the buttocks (Fig. 22.10). However, in general, forced-air warming is associated with a trend to a lower incidence of intraoperative pressure ulcers [283].

Risk of surgical site infections

Surgeons are sometimes concerned that the use of forced-air warming devices may increase the risk of surgical site infections. There are two potential problems associated with the use of forced-air warming devices. First, the devices can be contaminated with microbiological pathogens and second, forced-air warming may interfere with laminar air flow in some operating rooms.

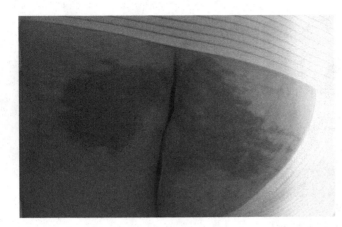

Fig. 22.10 Large full thickness pressure ulcer of the buttocks on the first postoperative day after complicated transapical aortic valve implantation with an underbody forced-air warming blanket.

Contamination of the devices

In general every device used in an operating room can be contaminated with microbiological pathogens coming from patients or from the staff working there. Therefore it is not surprising that several authors found that forced-air warming devices can be contaminated with microbiological pathogens [284–286], especially when the incorporated filters are not changed regularly according to the recommendations of the manufacturer [285, 286]. Micro-biological pathogens could be found at the nozzle where the device is usually touched by the operator [285, 286]. There is also sometimes contamination of the filters [285, 287] or other parts inside the power unit [286] and this can lead to microbes in the air flow going inside the forced-air warmer blanket [285, 286] despite the filter [284]. However, when a blanket is attached to contaminated devices no organisms grow on plates placed under the blanket [285].

Forced-air warming blankets are usually delivered clean, but not sterile, and therefore it is possible to find bacteria on the blanket prior to use. After using the blanket, more sites on the blanket are contaminated with bacteria. Therefore, once-used blankets should be not be reused with another patient.

Observations from volunteer studies

In a volunteer study no difference in the number of bacterial colonies on culture plates placed on the abdomen could be observed between a control period and a warming period of 2 hours, even though the skin of the volunteers was not disinfected [288]. In another study with volunteer patients with psoriasis with high shedding of skin in a laminar air flow theatre there was also no difference in the bacterial counts in a simulated operating field, although once again the skin of the volunteers was not disinfected [289].

Observations from patient studies

A clinical study with only four patients showed that use of forced-air warmers on patients produced a small increase in the number of colony forming units in air samples taken in the operative field, but the levels were estimated to be unlikely to have clinical significance. By far a greater effect on the number of colony forming units appeared to be the presence of the patient and staff in the theatre. During prolonged vascular surgery and hip arthroplasty [290], no risk for infection by forced-air warmers could be found. However, both studies were very small. In a retrospective data analysis of patients undergoing primary hip and knee replacement, no significant difference between forced-air warming and conductive warming for surgical site infection risk was found; however, the risk of developing deep infection was significantly higher in patients treated with forced-air warming. The study is very ambiguous because the authors state that record-keeping was incomplete for the additional risk factors that have already been identified as important predictors for deep infections. Additionally there was not only a change in the warming method during the study period, but also a change in the prophylactic antibiotic regimen [291]. There is concern that forced-air warming systems could increase bacterial contamination of the surgical wound and therefore some investigators advocate that forced-air warming systems should only be activated after the patient has been completely draped. This practice has no empiric support and puts the patient at an increased risk for hypothermia and surgical site infections [292].

In conclusion, forced-air warmers can be contaminated by microbiological pathogens, especially when the incorporated filters are not changed regularly. Nevertheless, to date no study could prove an increase in bacterial count or a higher infection rate with the use of forced-air warmers. In addition, the use of forced-air warmers to maintain normothermia is associated with a reduced risk of surgical site infection [168, 192].

Interference with laminar air flow

Laminar air flow or ultra-clean ventilation works by reducing the quantity of airborne bacteria in the operating theatre and at the surgical site. This goal is achieved by delivery of highly filtered air downwards with uniform velocity of about 0.3 to 0.5 m s^{-1}. As an undesired side effect, this high air velocity increases convective heat losses [276] and increases the risk of perioperative hypothermia [293]. Several studies found that laminar air flow can be disrupted when forced-air warming is used because the air flow and heat generated by the devices may lead to an ascending movement of the air [291, 294, 295]. This can increase the particle count above a simulated surgical site. However, sometimes these particles were artificially created and it is important to state that particle counts are not bacteria counts. In contrast, Sessler *et al.* found, in a more extensive study, that there was no reduction of operating room air quality during laminar flow ventilation when forced-air warming was used and therefore forced-air warming should remain an appropriate intraoperative warming method in laminar air flow theatres [296]. All these studies have the problem that they are using model situations with manikins. In a working operating theatre there are many people walking around, and surgical activity especially during orthopaedic surgery will surely disrupt laminar air flow even more.

Forced-air warmers may contaminate ultra-clean air ventilation; however, to date there is no definite link to an increased risk of surgical site infections [297, 298].

Increase in the environmental temperature

Forced-air warmers increase the temperature of the environment close to the patient, which is the workplace of anaesthesiologists and surgeons [294, 299]. Some operating room staff members may find this uncomfortable.

Falsely increased bispectral (BIS) index values

The BIS index is an electroencephalogram-derived index that is frequently used to monitor the hypnotic component of anaesthesia. There are several case reports that found that the use of a forced-air warmer falsely increased BIS index values in a clinical relevant way. The reason for this phenomenon is unclear. One possible explanation is that the blanket touching the face of the patient can sometimes cause fine vibratory movements that are detected by the device as muscular or electroencephalographic activity. In one report the phenomenon disappeared after separating the plastic cover from the face.

Thermal softening of tracheal tubes

During forced-air warming, marked softening and kinking of a polyvinyl chloride tracheal tube was observed. This can cause ventilatory problems if it is not recognised.

Drug overdose from transdermal medications

Several medications can be administered transdermally, for example nitroglycerin or fentanyl. There are case reports that describe drug overdose from the transdermal patch that was caused by active warming with a forced-air warmer blanket of the skin directly above the transdermal patch.

> To avoid the problem of drug overdose from transdermal medications, several measures are possible:
> 1. Discontinuation of the transdermal medication and administration of the drug via an alternative route or application of the transdermal medication to a location that will not be warmed by the blanket.
> 2. Use of a warming blanket that warms parts of the body other than where the transdermal medication has been applied or insulate the transdermal medications from the warming blanket [300].

Noise

Forced-air warmers produce noise in the operating room which can disturb the concentration of the staff and can interfere with communication among the team [266]. Noise produced by the power units ranges between 51 and 58 dBA, which is a clearly perceptible difference.

Electromagnetic fields

Electronic devices produce electromagnetic waves. Extremely low-frequency electromagnetic fields are produced by alternating currents that have a frequency of 50 or 60 Hz and are considered to have harmful effects to humans. In one study, extremely low-frequency electromagnetic fields from a forced-air warmer were higher than recommended by a Swedish TCO guideline within 30 cm. The authors therefore recommend that medical personnel and patients should establish sufficient distance from the device to be safe.

Conductive warmers

23

Conductive warming of the body surface is the only relevant alternative to forced-air warming. The efficacy of both methods relies heavily on the area that is actively warmed [254].

History

In the 1950s, prevention of perioperative hypothermia in babies and children began with the use of conductive warming mattresses [11, 12]. These devices were then used in adults during vascular surgery in the 1960s. Major advances in conductive warming were then made at the turn of the millennium when conductive carbon-fibre heating blankets [301, 302], water warming garments [303, 304] or adhesive water mattresses [165] were developed and introduced into clinical practice.

Efficacy

Conductive warming can be a very useful method of preventing perioperative hypothermia and the devices have the advantage that they are quieter than forced-air warmers. However, the classic circulating water mattress is inferior to forced-air warming [255, 301, 302], whereas conductive carbon-fibre heating blankets are equally effective [301, 302] and water warming garments [304] or adhesive water mattresses are even more effective then forced-air warming. To understand the differences between these devices, a basic knowledge of the technology and the physical background of conductive warming is necessary.

Technology of conductive warmers

Water-circulating mattresses

These devices consist of a heating or cooling unit and a mattress. The mattress is connected to the heating or cooling unit via a hose and the heated or cooled water circulates through the mattress. The mattress exchanges heat with the patient's skin surface and can be placed under the patient [255, 276] or on top [305]; some machines can supply several mattresses [305].

Air-circulating mattresses

These devices consist of a heating or cooling unit and a mattress. The mattress that is placed under the patient is connected to the heating or cooling unit via two hoses and the heated or cooled air circulates through the mattress. The mattress exchanges heat with the patient's back.

Electric conductive mattresses or blankets

These devices consist of a controller that generates a low voltage current. The mattress or mattresses can be attached via a cable and generate heat through semi-conductive wires [103], a carbon fibre fabric [301, 302, 306] or a carbon-polymer material [299, 307]. The mattresses can be placed under the patient [103, 308], on top [267, 301, 302, 306, 307] or even both.

Self-warming blankets

The blanket consists of several layers of polypropylene with integrated air activated warming pads. These pads are made up of air-permeable bags containing active coal, clay, salt, water and iron powder, and the pads create heat when the blanket is exposed to air by a chemical reaction with oxygen. The blanket is placed over the patient [309]. To date this is not sufficiently effective [309].

Water warming garments and adhesive water mattresses

These devices also consist of a heating or cooling unit and a mattress. The heating or cooling unit is usually connected to a thermometer that measures core temperature and uses these readings to regulate the degree of warming or cooling. The warming garments or adhesive water mattresses are connected to the heating or cooling unit via several hoses and the heated or cooled water circulates through the warming garment [303] or adhesive mattresses. Different sizes and shapes are available to enable optimal placement.

Physical background of conductive warmers

The mattress, blanket, garment or pads are connected to the warming or cooling unit and distribute the heat to the covered body surface, thereby transferring heat by conduction. The physics of this heat exchange process can be described as:

$$\dot{Q} = h_k \Delta T A \tag{23.1}$$

where
$\dot{Q}$ = heat transfer [W]
h_K = heat exchange coefficient [W m^{-2} °C^{-1}]
ΔT = mean temperature gradient between the mattress, blanket, garment or pad and the body surface [°C]
A = heat exchange area [m^2]

The heat exchange coefficient h_K defines the efficiency of the conductive heat exchange between the mattress, blanket, garment or pad and the body surface. It can be determined in a manikin or in volunteers by measuring the heat flux per unit area with heat flux transducers and simultaneously measuring the temperature gradient between the device and the body surface over a range of temperature differences. The heat exchange coefficient is then calculated using linear regression analysis by the slope of heat exchange per unit area as a function of the blanket–surface temperature gradient (Fig. 23.1).

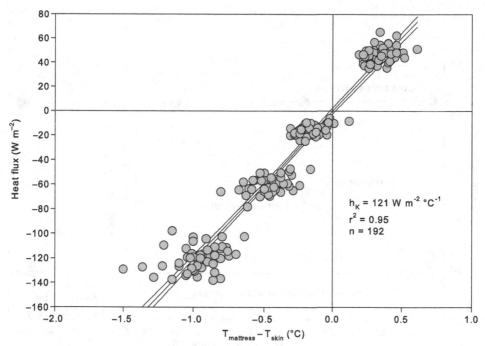

Fig. 23.1 Determination of the heat exchange coefficient for conduction (h_K) of a gel-coated water mattress. The slope of the regression line represents the heat exchange coefficient. Regression line and 95% confidence are shown. (Reproduced with permission from Wolters Kluwer: Bräuer A, Pacholik L, Perl T, English MJM, Weyland W and Braun U. Conductive heat exchange with a gel-coated circulating water mattress. Anesth Analg 2004; 99: 1742–1746 [52].)

The heat exchange coefficient for conduction warming is much higher than the heat exchange coefficient measured for forced-air warming. However, it is depending very much on the contact between the decice and the body surface. With older circulating water mattresses it was determined to be about 41 W m^{-2} °C^{-1} [275], whereas with a newer gel-coated water mattress or an adhesive water mattress it is between 110 and 121 W m^{-2} °C^{-1} [49, 52] because these mattresses have much closer contact with the skin.

It could be assumed that the high heat exchange coefficient guarantees a high heat transfer. However, this is not always the case because highly efficient heat exchange leads to fast warming of the skin thereby reducing the temperature gradient down to 0.3 °C [52] or 0.7 °C [276] and limiting heat transfer (Fig. 23.2). Another important factor is that the surface temperature of a mattress, blanket, garment or pad is lower than the temperature that is given by the warming or cooling unit. To enable heat transfer to the thermal core of the patient, the surface temperature of the mattress, blanket, garment or pad must be higher than the core temperature because according to the second law of thermodynamics, heat can flow only from higher to lower temperatures [52].

Similar to forced-air warming, the area that is used is of utmost importance for the resulting heat transfer. In contrast to forced-air warming, only the area of the skin that has direct contact with the warming device is of importance. This area is often smaller than expected, especially if the mattress, blanket, garment or pad is relatively stiff.

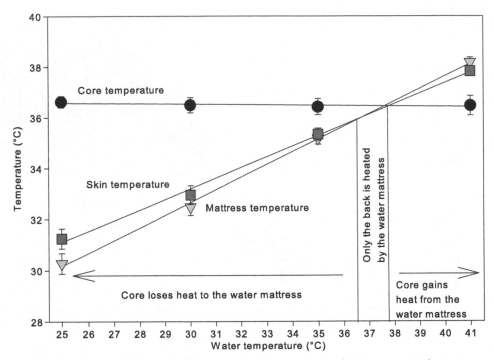

Fig. 23.2 Mattress temperature of a gel-coated circulating water mattress, skin temperature, and core temperature in relation to the water temperature of the warming or cooling unit. (Reproduced with permission from Wolters Kluwer: Bräuer A, Pacholik L, Perl T, English MJM, Weyland W and Braun U. Conductive heat exchange with a gel-coated circulating water mattress. Anesth Analg 2004; 99: 1742–1746 [52].)

Practical aspects

Conductive warming can be highly efficient if the contact of the mattress, blanket, garment or pad with the skin is good and enables a high heat exchange coefficient. The second important factor is the skin surface area that is in direct contact with the device. Additionally, if an area is warmed in which a large heat loss occurs without warming, then the effect is much better than if an area is warmed in which nearly no heat loss occurs like the back, because the impact on the heat balance is much smaller.

From these physical basics of heat transfer it can be expected that stiff water mattresses under the back of the body should not be very effective, because the contact is not very good, the area that is warmed is relatively small and the device warms in an area that normally does not lose very much heat. Normally the heat lost by a patient via the back is about 3 to 5 W [54] and the area is maximally 0.39 m². The calculated heat gain is a maximum of 11.2 W, which changes the heat balance at most by about 16 W. In a patient study a slightly smaller heat gain of 7 W and a change in the heat balance of 10 W was measured [54]. With the more effective gel-coated water mattress, which has closer contact with the skin and a higher heat exchange coefficient, the heat gain can be calculated to be about 18.4 W, which changes the heat balance about 23 W [52]. This change in the heat balance cannot stabilise the heat balance and therefore a conductive warming mattress under the back is not sufficient as a sole measure [54]. This is the main reason why these devices are inferior to forced-air warming [54, 166, 255, 301, 302, 310].

> Warming mattresses under the back of the body cannot be very effective.

In contrast, from the physical basics it can be assumed that conductive warming with warming mattresses or blankets that are placed on top of the body have a roughly comparable efficacy to forced-air warming blankets of the same size. Most of the studies have shown that conductive warming is comparably effective to forced-air warming when the same area is warmed [299, 301, 302, 311, 312], although some studies found a slightly better [306] or inferior efficacy [307].

> Conductive warming with warming mattresses or blankets that are placed on top of the body has a roughly equal efficacy to forced-air warming blankets.

Water warming garments or adhesive water mattresses have a high heat exchange coefficient due to the close contact with the skin, and cover a large area. Therefore they should be very effective and this has been shown in several studies [165, 303, 304, 313–315] and a meta-analysis [316]. However, the devices are very expensive [317] and are only cost effective in some selected cases [165].

> Water warming garments or adhesive water mattresses are extremely effective, but also extremely expensive.

Potential problems of conductive warming

Inadequate warming power

As stated earlier, conductive warming mattresses under the back cannot lead to a stable heat balance and therefore are not sufficient as a sole measure (Fig. 23.3) [54, 166, 255, 301, 302, 310].

The effect of conductive warming via the back can be improved when it is also used for prewarming [103, 308], in combination with good insulation in low-risk patients [103]. A sensible application of conductive warming mattresses under the back is their use in addition to forced-air warming because then the conductive warming mattress further improves the heat balance [183, 318].

Risk of burns

The risk of burns during conductive warming has been studied extensively and depends on several factors:

- The specific heat of the warming material [319]
- The temperature of the warming material [319]

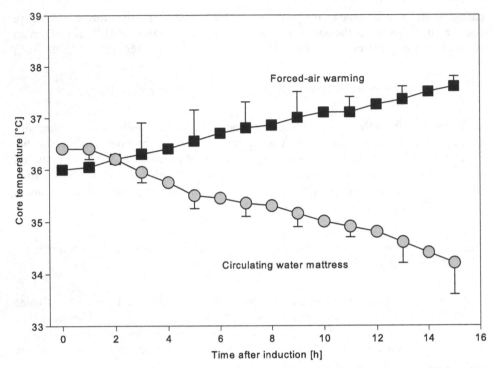

Fig. 23.3 Core temperature of adult patients during prolonged maxillofacial surgery warmed with forced-air warming (n = 8) or circulating water mattress under the back (n = 8). (Redrawn and modified using data from [255].)

- The heat capacity of the skin or the ability to absorb the heat
- The thermal conductivity of the skin or the ability to transport the heat [319]
- The thickness of the epidermis, dermis, fat and muscle [319]
- The blood flow through the different layers of skin [319]
- The appearance of oedema fluid [319]
- The duration of heat exposure [320].

There is a reciprocal relationship between the intensity of a thermal exposure and the amount of time required to produce a burn. Below a skin temperature of 43 °C more than 5 hours of warming are necessary to produce a burn (Fig. 23.4) [320]. This means that a temperature of 43 °C can be assumed to be safe.

However, there is only a small difference of about 0.5 °C between the skin temperatures that cause superficial first-degree burns and severe second- and third-degree burns [320]. This finding is of utmost importance because it means that there is almost no safety margin between a first-degree burn and a third-degree burn. And there is another reason for concern. These data were collected with pressure-free conductive warming [320]. The combination of pressure and heat can increase the risk of burns [82] and pressure ulcers.

The first reports of burns with circulating water mattresses date from the 1960s [321] and several horrible cases have been described, especially after malfunction of the devices (Figs. 23.5 and 23.6) [322–324].

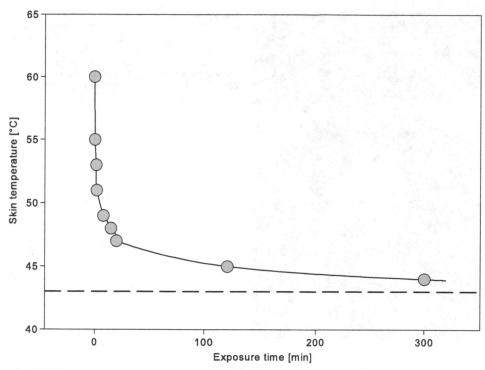

Fig. 23.4 Relationship of exposure time and skin temperature to cause a first-degree burn by conductive warming. The assumed safe limit of a skin temperature of 43 °C is symbolised by the dashed line. (Redrawn and modified using data from [320].)

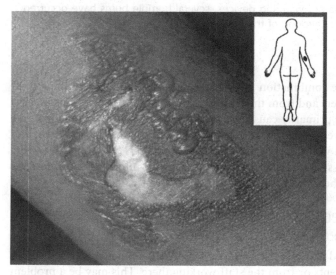

Fig. 23.5 Third-degree burn of the right elbow of a 9-year-old boy who underwent dental extraction. The injury was seen immediately after the 90 min procedure. The burn required subsequent split skin grafting and scar management. (Reproduced from Dewar DJ, Fraser JF, Choo KL, Kimble RM. Thermal injuries in three children caused by an electrical warming mattress. Br J Anaesth 2004; **93**: 586–589 by permission of Oxford University Press [323].)

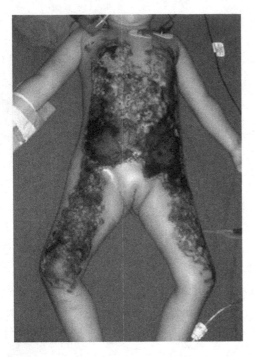

Fig. 23.6 Third-degree burn of a 3-year-old girl during the course of neurosurgical procedure. As a result of a malfunctioning device, a large full-skin burn occurred. (Reprinted from Acikel C, Kale B, Celikoz B. Major thermal burn due to intraoperative heating blanket malfunction. Burns 2002; **28**: 283–284 with permission of Elsevier [324].)

There has also been a case report of a burn that occurred with the use of a new warming garment [325].

> Conductive warming can lead to burns through the combination of heat and pressure. Especially due to malfunction of warming devices, several horrible burns have occurred and this necessitates regular checking of the devices.

Pressure ulcers

As already stated above, the combination of pressure and heat can increase the risk of burns [82] and pressure ulcers and from the clinical appearance it often remains unclear whether the skin lesion was primarily caused by heat, pressure or both. Many burn-like injuries are not burns but pressure ulcers. In a swine model, necrosis of muscle tissue can appear under pressure even when the warming surface is only 35 °C. Important factors that are responsible for pressure ulcers are pressure at bony prominences that interferes with the local circulation, shear forces and friction.

Risk of surgical site infections
Contamination of the devices

In general, every device used in an operating room can be contaminated with microbiological pathogens from patients or from the staff working there. This may be a problem with reusable mattresses. However, to date there have been no reports that this is really a problem. Water baths warming circulating water mattresses may be contaminated with bacteria and the contaminated fluid may spill in the operating room when the mattresses are connected and disconnected. While bacterial contamination of water baths of fluid warmers [326] and heat exchangers of cardiopulmonary bypass have been described no reports are available for heating or cooling units for circulating water mattresses.

Interference with laminar air flow

In contrast to forced-air warming, less interference with laminar air flow was observed with conductive warming devices [291, 294, 295]. It is unclear if this finding is of clinical relevance.

Chapter

24

Infusion warmers

Infusion warmers can be used to warm infusions and blood products. As the temperature of these products is usually below the core temperature of the body they can cause significant heat loss and lead to perioperative hypothermia, depending on the amount of fluid given [82].

History

In the 1950, severe perioperative hypothermia was recognised as a cause of intraoperative death during massive transfusions [2]. Therefore blood- and infusion-warming devices were one of the first measures against perioperative hypothermia.

Technology of infusion warmers

Fluid warmers are designed to deliver fluid at around body temperature to maintain perioperative normothermia. An infusion warmer should warm the fluid at the end of the tubing, where an intravenous cannula would be attached, to at least 33 °C to be effective. Several different technologies are used to achieve effective fluid warming. Most infusion warmers require a device-specific administration set. Each of these technologies has its own advantages and drawbacks.

Plate warmers

Plate warmers heat one or two metal plates of a special designed administration unit to warm the fluid, for example 3M Ranger 245, Belmont Buddy, Belmont Buddy lite, Biegler Protherm II, Estill Medical Technologies, Inc. Thermal Angel, Gaymar Medi-Temp III REF FW 600 Series Blood/Fluid warmer, JMW Medical Ltd Thermofluid TF251, Tyco Warmflo FW537-IB/System HEC40, Productions Hospitalièns Fancaises Gamida RSLB 30 H [327, 328].

Advantages: The shape of the administration set creates a large area for heat exchange.

Drawbacks: Leakage of the administration set is possible.

Drum warmers

Drum warmers heat a cylindrical or cone-shaped metal drum, and corresponding infusion tubing is wound several times around grooves in the drum to warm the fluid, for example Biegler BW 685, Biegler BW 685 S, Nuova/05, Nuova/05plus, Nuova/05plus W/0, Sarstedt Sahara Inline, Stihler Electronic GmbH Astotherm plus AP 220/220S/206/206S, Biotest Pharma GmbH BW385LB [328].

Advantages: No expensive administration set required.

Drawbacks: It is cumbersome and time-consuming to set up.

Counter-current warmers

Counter-current warmers heat a circulating fluid that flows in the opposite direction to the infusion fluid in a separate tube or channel, for example Smiths Level 1® H1200 Fast Flow Fluid Warmer, Smiths Hotline Blood and Infusion Warmer, Smiths Hotline Blood and Infusion Warmer 2.

Drawbacks: There is a small risk of the infusion tubing being damaged and that contamination of the infusion fluid can occur [326, 329].

Induction warmers

Induction warmers induce heat in a metal component of the administration set by an electromagnetic field, for example Belmont Rapid Infuser FMS 2000, Vital Signs enFlow IV Fluid/Blood Warming System, 37° Company Fluido® compact.

Drawbacks: Induction warmers should be placed more than 15 cm away from cardiac pacemakers or implantable cardioverters defibrillators (ICD) to avoid problems caused by the electromagnetic field.

Infrared warmers

Infrared warmers use halogen lamps to warm the infusion fluid by infrared radiation, for example TSCI Fluido.

Warm-air warmers

Warm-air warmers warm the infusion fluid with a special administration set in the hose of a forced-air warmer, for example BairHugger 241.

Advantages: No additional warming device necessary if a forced-air warmer is used.

Sleeve on infusion-tubing warmers

Sleeve on infusion-tubing warmers warm the infusion fluid via a heated sleeve around the patient line, for example Stihler Electronic GmBH Astoflo plus, Labor Technik Barkey GmbH & Co Autoline® [327, 328].

Advantages: Normal infusion tubing can be used. Sleeve on infusion-tubing warmers can also be used to keep the infusion fluid warm between another fluid warming device and the end of the tubing.

Drawbacks: Sleeve on infusion-tubing warmers are only effective at low flow rates.

Warming cabinets to prewarm fluids

Warming cabinets can be used to prewarm fluids before administration [330].

Advantages: Normal infusion tubing can be used.

Drawbacks: Warming time for the infusions is long. Only effective at high flow rates [327].

Table 24.1 Calculated heat loss induced by unwarmed infusions at different flow rates

Flow rate (ml h^{-1})	Heat loss (W)
100	1.6
500	8.1
1000	16.3
2000	32.6

Physical background of infusion warmers

The heat loss caused by cold or inadequate warmed infusions can be approximated by the following equation:

$$H = M \left(T_{Patient} - T_{Infusion}\right) c_{Infusion} \tag{24.1}$$

where

H = heat loss [kJ]

M = mass infused [kg]

$T_{Patient}$ = mean temperature of the patient [°C] (which is about 35 °C in a normothermic patient)

$T_{Infusion}$ = temperature of the infusion [°C]

$c_{Infusion}$ = specific heat of the infusion or blood product [kJ kg^{-1} °C^{-1}] [331].

To make it simple 1 l of infusion fluid weights nearly 1 kg and the specific heat capacity of a typical crystalloid fluid is about 4.19 kJ kg^{-1} °C^{-1}. Plasma has a slightly lower specific heat capacity (3.93 kJ kg^{-1} °C^{-1}) compared to crystalloid infusions and packed red blood cells have even lower specific heat capacity (3.22 kJ kg^{-1} °C^{-1}).

Heat loss induced by the infusion of unwarmed crystalloid fluid gives the results shown in Table 24.1.

If heat loss is calculated as the loss of mean body temperature, the following relationships can be found for a 70 kg patient with a metabolic rate of 93 W in an operating room with a room temperature of 21 °C (Fig. 24.1).

One litre of crystalloid solution administered at room temperature decreases mean body temperature by approximately 0.25 °C [82]. The influence of cold blood products infused at 4 °C is much more important, whereas with an effective infusion warmer warming the fluid or blood product to at least 33 °C, the temperature drop is minimal, even if high amounts of fluid have to be administered. However, it is also clear that warming an infusion up to 38 °C is not an effective way of raising the mean body temperature [82, 331].

Practical aspects

Most fluid warmers are designed for normal surgical patients and are effective up to flow rates of more than 3 l h^{-1} [327, 328, 331, 332]. Some fluid warmers are useful for paediatric surgery, whereas other infusion warmers are specially designed for surgery with very high blood loss and a large requirement for fluids and blood products [331, 333].

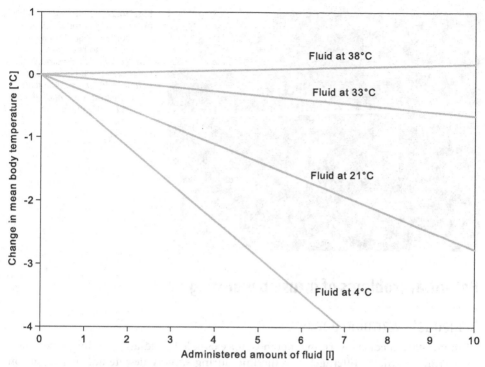

Fig. 24.1 Change in mean body temperature according to the quantity of administered fluid at different fluid temperatures. (Drawn using data from [83].)

It is sensible to place the fluid warmer close to the patient because a long distance between the heat exchanger and the end of the tubing can lead to significant heat loss [327], especially at lower flow rates and low room temperatures. Infusion warming is helpful to keep patients warmer [180, 334, 335], but without other adequate warming methods patients often get hypothermic during surgery, which is logical when the physical basis of infusion warming is kept in mind.

Infusion warmers minimise heat losses from the infusion of unwarmed fluids and cold blood products, and should be used when large amounts of intravenous fluid or blood are administered. However, infusion warming is not a substitute for adequate cutaneous warming and alone will not keep patients normothermic [82].

But how large an amount of fluid should lead to the use of an infusion-warming device? The NICE Guidelines recommend infusion warming when more than 500 ml of fluid will be given [17]. Horowitz *et al.* [332] recommended infusion warming when the administration of unwarmed fluids will lead to a drop in the mean body temperature of 0.5 °C to 1.0 °C, which would be equal to about 1000 to 2000 ml of fluid, whereas the German and Austrian guidelines recommend infusion warming at flow rates higher than 500 ml h^{-1} [20].

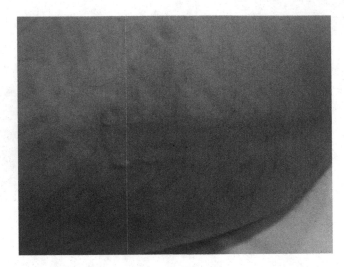

Fig. 24.2 Superficial skin burn over the deltoid muscle where the counter-current infusion warmer tubing had been in contact with skin. (Reproduced from Arrandale L, Ng L. Superficial burn caused by a Hotline fluid warmer infusion set. *Anaesthesia* 2009; **64**: 101-with kind permission of John Wiley & Sons, Inc. [338].)

Potential problems of infusion warming

Inadequate warming power

Without other adequate warming methods, for example forced-air warming or conductive warming, patients often get hypothermic during surgery despite adequate infusion warming.

Risk of burns

Warming infusions to very high temperatures can lead to full thickness burns and venous thrombosis [336]. There have been publications in which overheating of infusions or blood products exceeding 100 °C [337] with infusion warmers have been reported. This resulted in haemolysis and shock. Close contact of a counter-current infusion warmer to the skin has resulted in superficial burns of the skin with blistering (Fig. 24.2) [338].

Risk of infections

Every device in an operating room can be contaminated with microbiological pathogens from patients or from the staff working there. In water from counter-current warmers >100 000 colonies of multiple Gram-negative organisms have been found. Reports about infections caused by these devices are rare [331], but the presence of these organisms in infusion warmers is a potential threat, because during the disconnection of the administration set, contaminated water may spill out and contaminate the hands or gloves of the operator [329]. Leaks within counter-current infusion tubing have also been reported leading to mixing of the sterile infusion fluid and the non-sterile warming fluid [326, 339]. In addition to electrolyte disturbances and haemolysis this may lead to blood stream infection [339].

Air embolism

With increasing temperature, the solubility of gases in fluids or blood decreases and air bubbles containing mainly nitrogen will be created. Additionally, according to Charles's law, the volume of a gas is directly related to its temperature if the pressure is held constant. If an infusion fluid that normally contains small bubbles is heated, these bubbles will expand. This phenomenon is called outgassing [331] and is an inherent problem of infusion warming. Therefore, gas bubbles in the infusion fluid can frequently be seen with the use of infusion warmers. The air filters or bubble traps incorporated in some administration sets have only limited efficacy. However, the process of outgassing also occurs without infusion warming, inside the body; the only difference is that it is not visible to us.

Even if only small amounts of air will be infused, air bubbles can be trapped in the pulmonary arterial branches and platelets may aggregate on the air–blood interface of pulmonary arterial vessels, causing microthrombi. These small air emboli are often not associated with clinical problems; however, patients with patent foramen ovale may be at risk of air embolism to cerebral or other systemic arteries.

Chapter

25

Warming of irrigation fluids

In some endoscopic surgeries, such as transurethral resection of the prostate, large quantities of irrigation fluid are used to create a visual space and to clear the operating field from blood and cut tissue. If irrigation fluid is used at room temperature it contributes to the development of perioperative hypothermia [334, 340]. The effect is even more important when significant amounts of irrigation fluid are absorbed into the veins [340].

Warming of irrigation fluid during transurethral resection of the prostate

Transurethral resection of the prostate is a typical operation where large quantities of irrigation fluid are used and absorbed. The amount of irrigation fluid used ranges somewhat between 7 and 63 l [119, 341, 342]. Warming of this fluid leads to significantly higher core temperatures during and after the procedure [135] and less postoperative shivering. However, irrigation fluid is not the only source of heat loss during transurethral resection of the prostate and other warming measures are also necessary.

Arthroscopic surgery

Another type of operation where large quantities of irrigation fluid are used is arthroscopic surgery of the shoulder [343]. Most studies have found that irrigation fluid warming is helpful to maintain higher core temperatures [343]. In addition, local inflammatory response is significantly reduced by using warm irrigation fluid [343]. However, once again, irrigation fluid warming alone is not sufficient to prevent perioperative hypothermia in all patients.

Chapter

26

Insulation

Although some kind of insulation is used during every operation there is very little information about the properties of the various insulating materials used in the operating room. In general, insulation reduces heat losses from the skin [344] and thereby can help to achieve a stable heat balance. In contrast to other methods, insulation is a passive method that reduces heat losses to keep patients warm, but does not actively transfer heat.

Insulation materials

Insulation materials can be divided into two different types. The majority of insulation materials consist of so-called mass insulators that entrap air within a fibre matrix. Because this entrapped air does not move, it is called 'still air' or 'dead air', and is a very effective insulator. Therefore the insulation value of these materials is proportional to the thickness of the still air enclosed. The kind of fibre used to trap the air is of little importance [224, 344, 345]. The second type of insulation materials are so-called radiant insulators that are designed to reflect heat back to the radiating surface, emitting only a little radiant heat to the exterior. To provide a good effect, the radiant insulator should have a distance of about 1 cm from the radiating surface and this distance should consist of air. If this distance is filled by loose material of low bulk density, the effect of the radiant insulator is reduced [344].

Physical background of insulation

Theory of insulation

The heat exchange coefficient can be calculated from the heat flux per unit area and the temperature gradient between the surface and the environment. Covering a surface with insulation will decrease heat flux from the surface to the environment, therefore lowering the heat exchange coefficient. The reciprocal of the heat exchange coefficient defines the resistance to heat exchange, or the insulation [344]. Insulation values can be expressed in SI units (°C m^2 W^{-1}) or in the more straightforward Clo units. One Clo is the insulation that is required to keep a seated subject comfortable at an air temperature of 21 °C in an air movement of 0.1 m s^{-1}. Such insulation is provided by an ordinary suit, with shirt, trousers etc. and is equivalent to 0.155 °C m^2 W^{-1} [224].

When total insulation is calculated from the measured heat exchange coefficient h the following relationship exists:

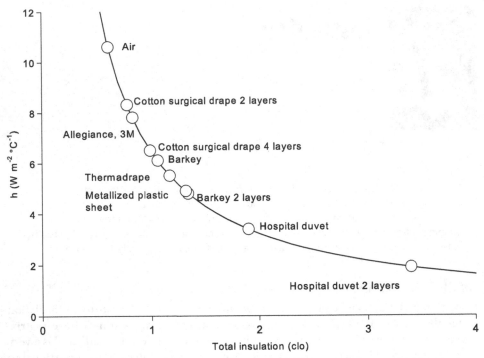

Fig. 26.1 Heat exchange coefficient values vs. total insulation of different insulation materials. There is a reciprocal relationship between the heat exchange coefficient and the total insulation. (Reproduced from: Bräuer A, Perl T, Uyanik Z, English MJM, Weyland W and Braun U. Perioperative thermal insulation: Only little clinically important differences? Br J Anaesth 2004; **92**: 836–840 [344] by permission of Oxford University Press.)

$$\text{Total insulation} = 6.45\,h^{-1} \qquad\qquad (26.1)$$

where

Total insulation = insulation of the material and insulation of air [Clo]

h = heat exchange coefficient [W m^{-2} °C^{-1}]

The insulation of air is about 0.6 Clo [48, 344]. The relationship between the heat exchange coefficient and the total insulation implies that adding a little insulation to an uninsulated surface decreases heat loss in a significant way (Fig. 26.1). Adding insulation to an already well-insulated surface cannot decrease heat loss very much if the temperature gradient between the surface and the environment does not change.

Practical aspects

Most commercially available insulation materials reduce heat loss by roughly 30% [346, 347]. The efficacy of these materials can be increased if more layers of the material are used [48]. The best available material designed for use in the operating room reduces heat loss from the covered area by about 45%, when used in two layers [344, 348].

Heat loss can be reduced significantly by insulation materials and therefore insulation should be applied to those areas of the body's surface that cannot be warmed actively. Insulation can only be effective when it is used to insulate a large body area. Clinical studies using mass insulators are very rare [349]. In contrast, radiant insulators have been studied extensively, with conflicting results. Some studies found that these insulators were effective in some special clinical situations [350, 351], whereas most others could not find any noteable efficacy [163, 352–354].

Potential problems of insulation

Inadequate efficacy

In a Cochrane meta-analysis [355], the benefit of extra thermal insulation compared with standard care is called into question. Clearly, passive insulation alone is insufficient to maintain normothermia, even in patients undergoing surgery with a low risk of hypothermia, like ENT surgery [103].

Inadequate thickness

Highly efficient mass insulators require sufficient thickness to provide adequate insulation. It was calculated that at least 1 cm thickness is needed to provide an insulation of 1.8 Clo.

Chapter

27

Radiative warmers

Radiative warmers use special bulbs or heated surfaces to generate infrared radiation. Radiative warming needs no contact between the warmer and the skin. However, in most perioperative situations radiative warming is cumbersome and has limited efficacy, and as a consequence the method is not very popular [82].

Physical background of radiative warming

Heat from radiative warmers is transferred by emission of electromagnetic radiation of infrared wavelength [48]. When the infrared electromagnetic radiation strikes the skin it is absorbed entirely because the emissivity of the human skin is about 0.98 [48, 224]. Radiative heat transfer is cumbersome to calculate, but some simple rules of thumb can help to use radiative warmers sensibly.

1. The energy of infrared electromagnetic radiation depends on the wavelength. The wavelength of infrared electromagnetic radiation ranges from 0.76 to 1000 µm and can be divided into three bands. These bands are usually called infrared-A (IR-A with a wavelength from 0.76 to 1.4 µm), infrared-B (IR-B with a wavelength from 1.4 to 3 µm) and infrared-C (IR-C with a wavelength from 3 to 1000 µm). The shorter the wavelength, the more energy can be transferred. That means that IR-A can transfer more heat than IR-C.

2. The penetration depth of infrared electromagnetic radiation also depends on the wavelength of the infrared electromagnetic radiation. The shorter the wavelength and higher the energy, the deeper the penetration into the skin.

3. Radiative heat transfer diminishes as a function of distance. This effect can be reduced somewhat by using parabolic-shaped reflectors like radiant ceilings [82].

4. Radiative heat transfer also decreases when the warming surface and the skin surface are not parallel to each other [82]. The best heat transfer occurs when the radiative beam strikes the skin perpendicularly. If the angle between the beam and the skin is less than 90°, the efficacy of heat transfer decreases rapidly.

5. Radiative heat transfer depends essentially on the area that is warmed. The larger the warmed area, the larger the heat transfer.

6. Insulation like blankets or clothing between the radiative warmer and the skin reduces the efficacy of radiative heat transfer.

Practical aspects

Radiative warming can be used for prewarming, intraoperative warming [51, 356] and postoperative rewarming of patients [50, 357, 358].

Radiative warming can be especially helpful during preparation for paediatric surgery, where hypothermia occurs quite often during induction of anaesthesia and insertion of intravascular catheters [82]. There are only a few trials that have studied the efficacy of radiative warmers during surgery and these studies have shown a limited efficacy [51, 356]. More studies have been conducted in the postoperative setting, where radiative warming was effective in preventing postoperative shivering [357, 358] and rewarming patients [50, 357, 358].

Advantages of radiative warming

Radiative warming can be a substitute for uncomfortably high ambient temperatures during preparation for paediatric surgery [82]. It may also be useful during trauma resuscitations because diagnostic and therapeutic manoeuvres restrict application of other active warming systems like forced-air warming [82].

Potential problems of radiative warming

Inadequate efficacy

A major limitation of radiant warming is that convective heat losses continue even during radiant warming. Together with the other restrictions, like a small available area for radiative warming this limitation makes the method relatively ineffective [82]. Furthermore radiative warming leads to heat stress in the vicinity of the warmer and therefore for the whole surgical team.

Chapter

28

Airway heating and humidification

Heat losses from the airways are of minor importance. Therefore it is not surprising that studies of active airway heating and humidification found that warming of inspiratory gases contributes little to preserve core temperature. The same is true for passive heat- and moisture-exchanging filters [82].

Physical background of airway heating and humidification

Heat loss from the airways can be divided in convective heat loss and evaporative heat loss. These are of minor importance compared to the heat loss from the skin. Model calculations and measurements from patients show consistently that heat loss from the airways is only about 7–10 W [56] with the convective heat loss being about 1 W and the evaporative heat loss about 6 W [56]. Heat- and moisture-exchanging filters (HME) retain significant amounts of moisture and heat within the respiratory system and reduce evaporative heat loss from the airways significantly [82]. In contrast, active airway heating and humidification aims to actively transfer heat to the body. However, the maximal air temperature is limited to prevent thermal injury of the airways. As a result, the influence of respiratory gas heating and humidification remains trivial because the total amount of heat transferred is so small [82]. This means that airway heating and humidification does not change the heat balance of the body very much and therefore has no relevant effect to prevent perioperative hypothermia [54].

Practical aspects

The small benefit of airway heating and humidification or heat- and moisture-exchanging filters observed in some clinical studies [359–361] probably results from erroneously warmed temperature probes positioned orally [360], in the nasopharynx or upper oesophagus [360] or insufficient randomisation [359]. In small infants, airway heating and humidification or heat- and moisture-exchanging filters may provide a small benefit in the prevention of perioperative hypothermia [182, 362] because of the higher alveolar ventilation and respiratory rate of small infants. In contrast, new devices combining active airway heating and humidification with infusion warming seem to be effective mainly because of the infusion warming [363].

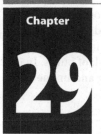

Chapter

Oesophageal warmers, negative-pressure warmers and endovascular warming catheters

Oesophageal warmers

> Oesophageal warmers have been used in several studies. However, due to the small heat exchange surface the devices are not effective [364].

Oesophageal warming actively transfers heat from a circulating water-perfused balloon placed in the oesophagus to the oesophageal mucosa. Even though conductive warming with good contact between the warmer and the warmed surface is very effective, the area that is warmed is extremely small. In one of the devices [365] it was about 0.042 m^2 [364]. It is impossible to transfer a large amount of heat through such a small surface without inducing a risk of thermal injury, even if in clinical studies some authors have found that the devices were efficient [365] or partially efficient. However, several other studies could not find any effect of oesophageal warming [366].

Negative-pressure warmers

> Negative-pressure warmers have been used in several studies. However, due to the small heat exchange surface the devices are not effective.

In recent years several negative-pressure warming devices have been developed and evaluated [367, 368]. These devices aim to overcome the restrictions of thermoregulatory vasoconstriction that reduces heat transfer from the periphery of the body to the core of the body [369] by mechanically distending blood vessels [367]. The theory is that mechanical vasodilation of subcutaneous venous plexuses will allow an extremely high blood flow through these areas and that heat applied to the skin can then be transferred freely to the core of the body. In the first study, hypothermic patients in the postanaesthetic care unit were rewarmed with the device at a rewarming rate of 13.6 °C h^{-1} [367], which is absolutely implausible. Another negative-pressure warming device was used with success during laparotomies. However, several other reliable studies have shown that the devices have no real effect [370], although one study showed that the device was non-inferior to forced-air warming during abdominal surgery [368]. However, this study only shows that forced-air warming initiated after prepping and draping with a small upper-body blanket is an insufficient warming concept during abdominal surgery.

Negative-pressure warming devices try to transfer a lot of heat through a small area. The heat exchange between the warmer and the skin may be very good, because the two surfaces are brought into close contact by the negative pressure. However, it is not possible to transfer a lot of heat through a small surface without the risk of burns. In one study, two patients developed second-degree skin burns with blistering and in one of the patients it took several weeks to heal [368].

Endovascular warming catheters

Endovascular warming catheters have been used in some selected patient groups with a high risk of perioperative hypothermia, with some success. However, the devices are very expensive [317].

Endovascular catheters that are usually used to induce and maintain therapeutic hypothermia have also been used to maintain normothermia during surgery. The control unit of the device circulates saline through balloons on the intravascular surface of the catheter that is usually placed in the femoral vein [371]. These devices have been used in patients undergoing burn surgery [371], trauma resuscitation [372] or off-pump coronary artery bypass surgery [317] with success. However, the devices are very expensive [317] and there have been several case reports about deep venous thrombosis associated with their use [373].

Chapter

30

Augmentation of heat production by amino acids or fructose

Preoperative administration of amino acids

> Preoperative administration of amino acids can increase metabolic heat production by a modest but clinically important amount [82], which can help to keep patients warmer.

In addition to increased metabolic heat production [374–377], the infusion of amino acids leads to the release of insulin and leptin. These hormonal signalling pathways may contribute to the thermogenic effect as well as having a modest influence on central thermoregulation [376]. However, if amino acid infusion is started after the development of intraoperative hypothermia, this treatment fails to accelerate rewarming [378]. The administration of amino acids can increase cardiorespiratory demands and may cause a considerable challenge to elderly patients or patients with reduced cardiopulmonary reserve.

Preoperative administration of fructose

> Preoperative administration of fructose can also increase metabolic heat production [379].

In addition to increased metabolic heat production, the infusion of fructose leads to a modest influence on central thermoregulation [379]. However, in patients with undiagnosed hereditary fructose intolerance the infusion of fructose can cause death due to renal and liver damage.

> Preoperative administration of amino acids is an experimental option and is currently not recommended by guidelines. In contrast, preoperative administration of fructose can cause death in patients with undiagnosed hereditary fructose intolerance and should be avoided.

Modern perioperative temperature management

Modern perioperative temperature management aims at the reduction of postoperative morbidity. The key elements are implementation of a warming concept that includes measurement of core temperature, prewarming, warming therapy during anaesthesia and postoperative therapy for residual hypothermia (if existent) and shivering.

It is sensible to describe the perioperative temperature management in detail in a standard operating procedure as a part of quality management in anaesthesiology [380].

Core temperature measurement

Preoperative core temperature measurement is essential to detect patients with a low core temperature at this stage.

These patients benefit from intensified preoperative warming therapy. For that purpose sublingual temperature is the most suitable option [227, 245, 259]. Alternatively zero-heat-flux thermometers or double-sensor thermometers may be used. The use of infrared-thermometers is too inaccurate and should not be used unless better alternatives are not available [20].

Intraoperative core temperature measurement is essential to detect perioperative hypothermia, to control the effectiveness of warming therapy [230], to prevent overheating and to facilitate detection of malignant hyperthermia [32].

Therefore it is recommended by the ASA, the evidence-based guidelines for prevention of perioperative hypothermia of the Canadian Association of General Surgeons [19], the ASPAN Guidelines [18], the NICE Guidelines [17] and the German and Austrian Guidelines [20]. Ideally core temperature should be monitored continuously or at least every 15 minutes [20] and in all patients undergoing surgery that lasts longer than 1 hour [32] under general or neuraxial anaesthesia [20]. In patients under general anaesthesia, nasopharyngeal temperature measurement is the most suitable option due to its high accuracy and ease of use. Alternatively sublingual temperature, oesophageal temperature, bladder temperature, zero-heat-flux thermometers or double-sensor thermometers may be used. The use of infrared thermometers is too inaccurate and should not be used if better alternatives are available [20].

To avoid measurement errors the site of core temperature monitoring should be far away from the operative field.

Postoperative core temperature measurement is essential to detect postoperative hypothermia and to indicate postoperative warming therapy. For that purpose sublingual temperature is the most suitable option in awake patients. Alternatively bladder temperature (if available), zero-heat-flux thermometers or double-sensor thermometers may be used. The use of infrared-thermometers is too inaccurate and should not be used if better alternatives are available [20]. In sedated and ventilated patients, nasopharyngeal temperature, oesophageal temperature or bladder temperature can be used.

Prewarming

There are several studies showing clearly that the intraoperative use of forced-air warming without prewarming is often ineffective [140, 258]. Therefore prewarming is an essential part of modern perioperative thermal management.

Without prewarming, redistribution of heat after induction of anaesthesia often causes hypothermia [80]. This is especially true in patients with a low core temperature and a cold periphery before induction of anaesthesia.

Warming therapy during anaesthesia

During anaesthesia, forced-air warming or conductive warming are effective for most surgical procedures. During anaesthesia, the largest blanket or cover that is possible for the operation should be used. If significant amounts of intravenous fluids are used during the procedure, body-surface warming must be combined with adequate fluid warming [260].

Postoperative therapy of residual hypothermia and shivering

If patients are hypothermic when they arrive in the postanaesthetic care unit or intensive care unit [137–139], despite all preoperative and intraoperative measures, they should be actively rewarmed. Postanaesthetic shivering should be treated.

Chapter

32

Prewarming

Prewarming can be defined as active warming of the body surface before induction of anaesthesia or neuraxial anaesthesia. It is an essential part of modern perioperative temperature management and cannot be substituted by other measures.

In the previous chapter the combination of prewarming, warming during anaesthesia and infusion warming was recommended for modern perioperative temperature management. Is prevention of perioperative hypothermia really as simple as that? Yes, it is. A combination of these three elements enables postoperative hypothermia rates of less than 20%, even in large retrospective studies [381]. Prewarming is a key element of perioperative warming therapy [382] and cannot be substituted by intraoperative measures. The reason for this is that prewarming aims at the reduction of the initial drop in core temperature after induction of anaesthesia, which is caused by the redistribution of heat from the core of the body to the periphery [80]. In contrast, warming therapy during anaesthesia and infusion warming aim at maintaining or restoring a thermal balance during the operation, which is another mechanism of the development of perioperative hypothermia.

How does prewarming work?

Active warming of the body surface changes the heat balance of the body dramatically and increases the heat content of the peripheral tissues.

The skin under a warming blanket is no longer a source of heat loss but a source of heat gain [260]. Normally, heat flows from the core of the body to the periphery and then to the environment. This is changed during prewarming. The heat that is produced in the core of the body still flows to the periphery, but at the same time heat applied to the skin surface also flows into the peripheral tissues. These two mechanisms together lead to an increase in the heat content and temperature of the peripheral tissues [79]. The core temperature is only minimally influenced [79, 102, 383, 384].

After a long cooling period the heat content of the arms and the legs rises very fast during the first hour of prewarming and then reaches a plateau after 2 hours [79]. The time until the heat content of the peripheral tissues reaches a plateau is probably much shorter if the patient's periphery was not exposed to a cold environment for long. This is one of the reasons why even very short periods of prewarming are effective [102, 384].

Prewarming reduces the temperature gradient between the core and the periphery of the body. Because the redistribution of heat after induction of anaesthesia is directly proportional to the temperature gradient between the core and the periphery of the body, a small temperature gradient leads to a small redistribution of heat and thereby to a small decrease in core temperature after induction of anaesthesia. No other measure can do this. The prevention of this initial drop in core temperature is very important, because many patients arrive with a core temperature below 36.5 °C [61, 167] and because the highest rate of hypothermia can be observed after the first hour of anaesthesia [140] which is a consequence of the redistribution of heat.

The efficacy of prewarming has been shown in many volunteer studies [79, 116, 383], clinical studies [102, 129, 162, 256, 258, 312, 318, 341, 385–387], meta-analyses [388, 389] and retrospective studies [381]. A few studies did not show that prewarming is effective [309, 390], especially if a minor or minimally effective warming method was used [309]. Therefore prewarming is recommended in some guidelines [19, 20] as a routine measure. However, prewarming is still one of the most underutilised measures to prevent perioperative hypothermia [240].

Barriers against the use of prewarming

Prewarming is a very easy procedure. The patient just has to be warmed with a warming blanket and the corresponding power unit. No special equipment is necessary nor specially trained personel. However, the organisation of prewarming can be challenging, because the implementation of prewarming necessitates some changes in the daily routine. Typical barriers are:

1. Many physicians and nurses are not convinced that it is really necessary to change their daily practice that has been the standard for many years.
2. Many physicians and nurses are convinced that patients do not want active prewarming. This is not true, because prewarming increases the thermal comfort of patients [391] and only a few patients (<5%) refuse prewarming or stop prewarming because of intolerance to heat [384].
3. For several years many anaesthesiologists thought that duration of prewarming must be at least between 30 and 60 minutes [79]. It is true that it is extremely difficult to realise a prewarming period of 60 minutes for every patient without causing massive delays in the daily operating room (OR) schedule. However, a study by Horn et al. [102] showed that even 10 to 20 minutes of prewarming can be very efficient. This makes it much easier to realise a prewarming programme without leading to inefficiency in the perioperative processes.

To start a prewarming programme it is important to achieve a broad consensus between all staff working in the operating room that prewarming is a necessary and important part of the preoperative preparation of the patient for anaesthesia and surgery. This consensus is needed to overcome the barriers against prewarming and to find adequate solutions for all the minor problems that can and will occur during the implementation of prewarming. Without such a consensus and the clearly stated will to make prewarming an integral part of patient management it is very difficult to achieve a high prewarming rate.

Which patients should be prewarmed?

As already described, general anaesthesia [80] or neuraxial anaesthesia [81] leads to an initial drop in core temperature due to redistribution of heat. The only effective measure against this drop in core temperature is prewarming. Therefore it makes sense to prewarm every patient undergoing general anaesthesia with a duration of more than 30 min [20] and every patient undergoing neuraxial anaesthesia [20]. In patients undergoing short procedures, prewarming alone can be sufficient [20].

Where can prewarming be performed?

There is no single strategy that suits all hospitals and situations, but there are several locations where patients can be prewarmed: on the ward, in the preoperative holding area, in the induction room or in the OR if no induction room is available.

Prewarming on the ward

If prewarming is planned on the normal ward [258, 381] several prerequisites are required:

- Several forced-air warmers with warming gowns or several power units and warming mattresses must be available on the normal wards.
- There must be enough storage room available for the devices and the warming gowns and mattresses.
- Staff on the ward have to be trained that prewarming is now an integral part of the preoperative preparation.
- The patients have to be adequately informed about the benefits of prewarming.
- There must be reliable organisation of the OR schedule and timely informing of the ward about the time that the patient will be called into the OR.
- Patients must then immediately receive their warming mattress or warming gown to give enough time for prewarming.
- The same warming systems must be used on the ward and in the OR.
- The patient must be positioned on the OR table together with the warming gown or warming mattress.
- Responsibility for and organisation of cleaning and transportation of reusable warming mattresses must be clarified. This is not necessary when single-use gowns are used.

Prewarming in the holding area

Prewarming started on the ward can be continued in the holding area or can be started there [102, 259, 384]. Since patients usually stay for some time in the holding area, this waiting time can be used sensibly for prewarming. If prewarming is planned in the holding area, several prerequisites must be met to allow effective prewarming:

- The holding area must be large enough to allow parallel prewarming of several patients at the same time.
- There must be enough forced-air warmers with warming gowns or blankets available in the holding area.
- There must be sufficient storage room for the devices and the warming gowns or blankets.

- There must be reliable organisation to allow sufficient time for prewarming in the holding area.
- The staff in the holding area must be trained that prewarming is an integral part of the preoperative preparation.
- The patients have to be adequately informed about the benefits of prewarming.
- Prewarming must be started immediately after arrival of the patient in the holding area, because sometimes the stay in the holding area is unpredictably short.

Prewarming in the induction room or in the operating room

Prewarming started on the ward or in the holding area can be continued in the induction room or in the operating room when no induction room is available or it can be started there [256, 390, 392]. If prewarming is planned in the induction room or in the operating room the following prerequisites must be met:

- The induction room must be equipped with a forced-air warming power unit in addition to the forced-air warming power unit in the operating room itself.
- The placement of the power unit has to enable all routine measures without interference of the prewarming process.
- There must be reliable organisation to allow sufficient time for prewarming.
- Patients have to be adequately informed about the benefits of prewarming, either during the preoperative preparation or immediately before prewarming.
- The anaesthesia nurses must be trained that prewarming is an integral and important part of the preoperative preparation.
- Prewarming must be started immediately after arrival of the patient in the induction room, because there is not much time for prewarming.

Each of these possibilities has its advantages and disadvantages. The most important arguments are listed in Table 32.1.

In Germany more than 80% of the anaesthesiologists that prewarm their patients do so in the induction room, about 20% in the holding area and very few patients are prewarmed on the normal ward [240].

Prewarming in the induction room or in the operating room seems to be the most convenient setting. In addition it allows warming of the patient continuously through the induction period. However, prewarming in the holding area is also very effective.

Which blanket should be used?

From an economic standpoint it is sensible to use the same blanket for prewarming and for warming therapy during anaesthesia, because otherwise two warming blankets have to be used.

Most volunteer studies have used full-body blankets, because these blankets cover the largest body surface area [79, 383]. However, these blankets can only be used during some operations, for example ENT surgery. Therefore, many anaesthesiologists use

Table 32.1 Advantages and disadvantages of prewarming of different locations for prewarming

Prewarming on the ward

Advantages	Disadvantages
• Patients are prewarmed as soon as possible and further prewarming is possible in the holding area or in the induction room. • The use of the warming gown or warming mattress can be continued in the holding area or during the induction of anaesthesia and during the operation.	• The number of forced-air warming power units and warming gowns or power units and warming mattresses that are required is very high. • Many physicians and nurses on the wards have to be trained. • Prewarming means additional work for the staff on the ward and there is no control of the prewarming process by an anaesthesiologist.

Prewarming in the holding area

Advantages	Disadvantages
• The anaesthesiologist can have some control of the prewarming process. • The training of the staff in the holding area only requires a short time because the number of people that must be trained is small. • The number of forced-air warmers or power units used is low.	• Prewarming means additional work for the staff in the holding area. • Sometimes patients bypass the holding area and arrive in the OR without prewarming.

Prewarming in the induction room or in the operating room

Advantages	Disadvantages
• Prewarming in the induction room or operating room is very effective, because patients can also be warmed continuously during the whole induction period. • The anaesthesiologist has maximal control of the prewarming process. • Prewarming in this setting needs very little additional time. • Training of the nurses does not require much time, because the number of people that must be trained is small and the warming equipment is familiar to the staff.	• If prewarming in the induction room is the only prewarming measure and it fails, the patient cannot be prewarmed. • The number of forced-air warming power units that are required is high.

upper-body blankets that can be used during the operation. These blankets are turned to the long-axis of the patient for prewarming [129]. Another possibility is the use of lower-body blankets or underbody blankets which are frequently used in infants. In several studies with outpatients, warming gowns were used [391]. This makes particular sense in the ambulant setting because the use of warming gowns eliminates the need for other clothing and nearly all ambulant operations can be performed using warming gowns.

Which temperature setting should be used?

In an extremely well-controlled volunteer study there was no real difference in the efficacy of prewarming with a forced-air warmer set at 38 °C or at 43 °C [79]. However, there are some arguments for the use of a high temperature setting:

- The heat transfer is slightly higher [79].
- In the clinical setting time for prewarming is often very limited.
- If prewarming is used in the induction room or operating room and is continued throughout the whole duration of anaesthesia the risk of forgetting to increase the temperature setting after induction of anaesthesia is lower.
- There is no thermal discomfort with a high temperature setting during a short prewarming period [79].

> The highest temperature setting should be used during prewarming to achieve maximum efficacy. If the patient experiences thermal discomfort, the temperature setting should be lowered. It can be assumed that the patient is then vasodilated and the periphery is warm.

How long should patients be prewarmed?

> The best answer is probably: As long as possible, but at least 10 to 20 minutes.

In most countries time resources are limited by the high economic pressure on the health system. This makes it impossible to delay the next case to prolong prewarming. Therefore, prewarming on the normal ward or in the holding area has to be stopped when the patient is called into the operating room. Initially it was thought that the optimal prewarming time was 30 to 60 minutes [79]. However, a very well-performed clinical study showed that even 10 to 20 minutes is very effective [102] and is therefore recommended by the German and Austrian guidelines [20].

If prewarming is performed in the induction room or operating room the time available for prewarming can be maximised if prewarming is started as soon as the patient enters the room (Fig. 32.1). The patient is then getting prewarmed while the surgical safety checklist is ticked off (patient has confirmed identity, site, procedure and consent; the operation site is marked, the anaesthesia safety check completed and so on). After ECG monitoring, pulse oximeter and blood pressure measurement is attached to the patient and functioning, and an adequate intravenous access is established, about 10 minutes are usually gone. This is then the available prewarming time and is sufficient for many patients and procedures. If a thoracic epidural catheter is placed for large abdominal or thoracic procedures the prewarming time is even longer (Fig. 32.2).

Are there patients that should not be prewarmed?

In case of life-threatening emergencies that require immediate surgical intervention no prewarming is possible. However, even in these cases warming should be started as early as possible, because initiation of warming needs only about 1 minute of time and this

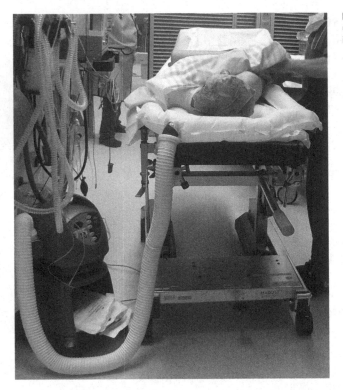

Fig. 32.1 Prewarming with an underbody blanket in the induction room.

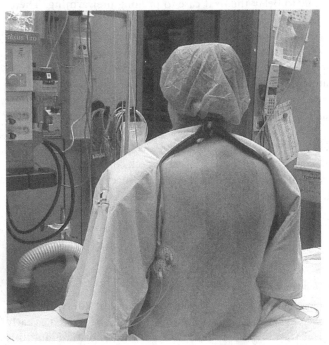

Fig. 32.2 Prewarming in the induction room immediately before insertion of a thoracic epidural catheter. (Photo by Marc Jipp).

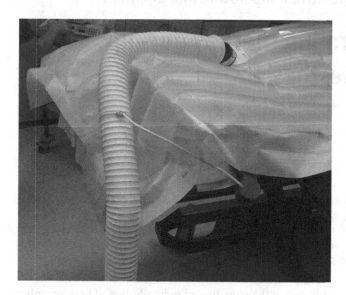

Fig. 32.3 Nozzle connected to the operating table with a clip to prevent the weight of the nozzle tearing the blanket from the patient.

time delay is very often no problem, even in emergencies, whereas deep perioperative hypothermia is associated with bad outcomes [138, 187].

To date no data are available that show significant risks due to prewarming. Patients undergoing surgery with peripheral nerve blocks or local anaesthesia without analgose-dation seem to have a very low risk of hypothermia and therefore probably do not need active warming therapy and prewarming. Infants and children undergoing magnetic resonance imaging under sedation can show an increase in core temperature and therefore probably need no prewarming [393]. Patients arriving in the operating room with fever also do not seem to need prewarming.

Practical tips and tricks

- The forced-air warming device should be placed near the wall or near the end of the operating table. This positioning normally allows all routine measures without interference.
- If it is not possible to warm the whole body with the prewarming blanket it is sensible to warm primarily the legs of the patient because during the redistribution of heat about 75% of the heat is distributed to the legs [79].
- The nozzle should also be connected to the blanket close to the legs because the air temperature in the warming blanket is higher there. This will increase heat flow to the legs.
- The nozzle should be connected to the operating table with a clip because otherwise the weight of the nozzle can tear the blanket from the patient (Fig. 32.3).
- There should be no blanket between the warming blanket and the patient.

Warming therapy during anaesthesia

Warming therapy during general and neuraxial anaesthesia is recommended by several guidelines [17, 20]. It is important to realise that the recommendation is to warm patients during anaesthesia and not only during surgery. This distinction is important because there is a relevant time delay between the induction of anaesthesia and the start of surgery, due to positioning, surgical skin preparation and waiting times.

In contrast to prewarming, which aims at the reduction of redistribution of heat, warming during anaesthesia and infusion warming aim at maintaining or restoring a thermal balance during anaesthesia and surgery, which is a different mechanism of development of perioperative hypothermia. If it is possible to start warming therapy at induction of anaesthesia it should also be possible to start it a few minutes earlier, so that prewarming continues into warming therapy during anaesthesia. It is not a problem to induce anaesthesia during warming therapy (Fig. 33.1). Epidural catheters, airway devices, arterial and central venous lines can be placed without any difficulty. Only if a bladder catheter has to be placed will some warming blankets have to be moved aside for a short time.

After induction of anaesthesia, positioning of the patient, surgical skin preparation and covering of the patient can be performed under active warming therapy. There is no related risk of increasing the particle and bacterial count due to warming, because the particle count of the air in the operating room is mainly determined by the number of people present [394] and not by the use of forced-air warmers [395]. If active warming must be stopped during surgical skin preparation this interruption should be as short as possible, because the already warmed skin then loses a lot of heat to the environment [383].

Which blanket should be used during anaesthesia?

There is an ever-increasing number of forced-air warming blankets on the market and not every type of blanket has been evaluated. As a rule of thumb the largest blanket possible during the planned operation should be used [270], because the area covered by the blanket is of utmost importance. The larger the area, the better the efficacy of the forced-air warming blanket. The reason for this is that forced-air warming blankets are not only transferring heat to the body. More important is the fact that they are reducing the heat losses from the covered area to zero. The fact that the skin under a forced-air warming blanket is no longer an important source of heat loss, but a source of heat gain, changes the heat balance of the body and is responsible for the observed higher efficacy of larger forced-air warming blankets [260]. However, during most operations the large full-body blankets

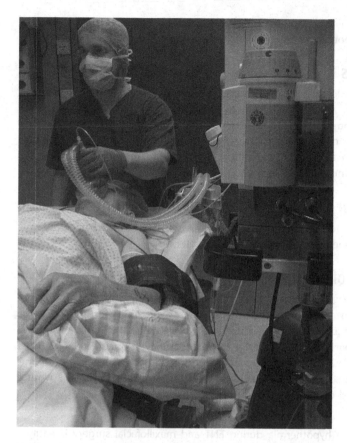

Fig. 33.1 Active warming therapy during induction of anaesthesia with an underbody blanket.

cannot be used. Therefore surgical access blankets, underbody blankets, lithotomy blankets, lower-body blankets or upper-body blankets have to be used.

During anaesthesia, core temperature should be monitored because it is possible to overheat patients during effective warming therapy, especially children [104, 272]. As a rule of thumb the temperature of forced-air warmers should be reduced to 34 °C if the core temperature exceeds 37.3 °C to prevent overheating.

A sensible alternative to forced-air warming is conductive warming with modern conductive warming devices, which are also effective in many settings [299, 301, 302].

Addition of infusion warming

Infusion warming is also recommended by several guidelines to prevent intraoperative hypothermia [17, 19, 20]. However, there are some differences in the guidelines as to when infusion warmers should be used in addition to forced-air warming. The NICE Guidelines, for example, recommend infusion warming when more than 500 ml of fluid will be given [17], whereas the German and Austrian guidelines recommend fluid warming when more than 500 ml h^{-1} is necessary [20]. The general idea of all guidelines is to recommend infusion warming when larger amounts of fluids are used, because then the infusion of cold fluids becomes an important source of heat loss.

Additional measures

Active surface warming and infusion warming are the mainstays for the prevention of perioperative hypothermia. Additional measures like conductive warming of the back with a heating mattress [166], insulation of the parts of the body that cannot be actively warmed [20], an adequate room temperature [20] and the use of heat and moisture exchangers can be used to further increase the efficacy of warming therapy, but the effects of these additional measures are not very large.

Warming therapy for different procedures and patients

In the next paragraphs some typical problems and possibilities to avoid perioperative hypothermia will be described without claim of completeness.

Head, neck and maxillofacial procedures

During intracerebral surgery it is relatively easy to maintain perioperative normothermia [396], because a large area of the body surface is available for warming therapy. The same is true for most ENT and maxillofacial procedures. However, without adequate warming therapy many patients experience perioperative hypothermia even during relative short procedures [96, 103, 309, 397] and even after ENT and maxillofacial surgery perioperative hypothermia can be associated with postoperative complications [398] like wound healing problems [206] and cardiac complications [399].

> Prevention of perioperative hypothermia during ENT and maxillofacial surgery is easily possible with whole-body blankets, lower-body blankets, torso blankets or underbody blankets that are used for prewarming and warming therapy during anaesthesia. In most cases an infusion warming system is not necessary.

Thoracic procedures

In a study of more than 2000 patients, about 50% of all patients were hypothermic after thoracic surgery [400]. Much better results can be achieved with the sequential use of prewarming and warming therapy during anaesthesia. This is very important because many patients are at risk of experiencing cardiac complications after thoracic surgery.

> Prevention of perioperative hypothermia during thoracic surgery is possible with lower-body blankets or underbody blankets that are used for prewarming and warming therapy during anaesthesia. An infusion warming system is especially necessary during oesophageal resections. It is challenging to keep patients normothermic during oesophageal resection.

Intra-abdominal procedures

Maintenance of normothermia during intra-abdominal procedures like colorectal surgery is of extreme importance to reduce postoperative complications [168]. Combined epidural and general anaesthesia are frequently used and have a high risk for the development of perioperative hypothermia. With a combination of prewarming, warming therapy during anaesthesia and fluid warming, hypothermia is rarely observed, even in these patients [129]. In general there is no difference in the risk of perioperative hypothermia between laparotomy and laparoscopy surgery [401–403]. Warming and humidification of insufflation gas during laparoscopic procedures is not very helpful in preventing hypothermia.

> Prevention of perioperative hypothermia during intra-abdominal surgery is possible with upper-body blankets, lower-body blankets, surgical access blankets, poncho blankets, lithotomy blankets or underbody blankets that are used for prewarming and warming therapy during anaesthesia. During many procedures an infusion warming system is necessary. It can be challenging to keep patients normothermic during extensive intra-abdominal procedures.

Orthopaedic surgery

Maintenance of normothermia during orthopaedic procedures like hip or knee arthroplasty is of importance to reduce blood loss in these patients [164, 170]. Without prewarming and without fluid warming about 25% to 30% of the patients become hypothermic [209].

> Prevention of perioperative hypothermia during orthopaedic procedures is possible with upper-body blankets, torso blankets, poncho blankets, lithotomy blankets or underbody blankets that are used for prewarming and warming therapy during anaesthesia. During many procedures an infusion warming system is necessary.

Caesarean section

To date, spinal anaesthesia is the most common method for caesarean section. Typically a height of block to T4 or T5 is achieved. This extensive blockade puts the patients at a higher risk of hypothermia [115]. In addition, due to preloading or co-loading with intravenous fluids and a vasopressor to minimise hypotension, patients undergoing caesarean section may receive large amounts of fluids during the operation [404]. Therefore maternal hypothermia is common during caesarean section, even when forced-air warming and/or fluids warming are used [404]. Both methods – forced-air warming [405] and fluid warming – are able to reduce the magnitude of decrease in core temperature [387, 404], but in some studies without prewarming the effect was not sufficient [406] and the incidence of perioperative hypothermia was still high [407].

Maternal hypothermia may contribute to neonatal hypothermia, which is associated with an increased likelihood for more severe early respiratory distress and mortality in the newborn [408]. However, neonatal hypothermia can also develop during intraoperative bonding, while the newborn is positioned on its mother's chest. This neonatal hypothermia can be prevented if bonding of the newborn takes place under the forced-air warming blanket that is used to keep the mother warm [405].

> Prevention of perioperative hypothermia during caesarean section can be performed with upper-body blankets, poncho blankets or lithotomy blankets that are used for prewarming

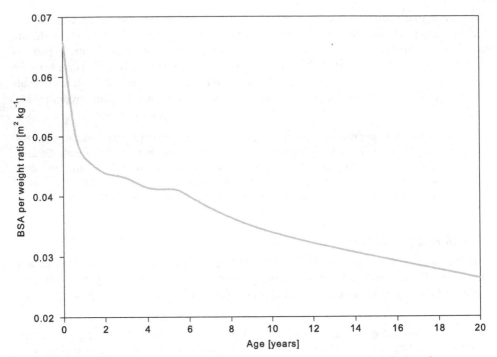

Fig. 33.2 Body surface area (BSA) to weight ratio vs. age in paediatric patients. A high body surface area to weight ratio increases the risk of perioperative hypothermia.

and warming therapy during anaesthesia. Additional infusion warming is necessary, but some patients will still experience hypothermia.

Maternal hypothermia can contribute to neonatal hypothermia, which can also develop during intraoperative bonding. This neonatal hypothermia can be prevented if bonding of the newborn takes place under the forced-air warming blanket that is used to keep the mother warm [405].

Paediatric procedures

Thermoregulation of paediatric patients is impaired by anaesthetics in the same way as it is in adults [91]. Compared to adults the head of a child is relatively large and the extremities are relatively small. As a consequence small children develop only a relatively small drop in core temperature after induction of anaesthesia, because the redistribution of heat to the extremities is limited. Therefore prewarming is not very successful in small children, but can be successful in older children undergoing spinal surgery [409].

However, during anaesthesia paediatric patients lose more heat to the environment than adults because cutaneous heat loss is roughly proportional to the body surface area, whereas metabolic heat production is roughly proportional to body mass (Fig. 33.2). As a consequence, infants and children cool faster than adults [410] and perioperative hypothermia rates can be high [411].

Because the body surface area is so large compared to the weight, newborns, infants and children can be warmed very well with forced-air warmers [410] if these devices cover a large area [104, 272]. In addition to forced-air warming, an ambient temperature of about 24 °C can be helpful to prevent hypothermia [20, 410].

> Prevention of perioperative hypothermia during paediatric procedures is usually conducted with underbody blankets. Therefore these blankets are almost automatically used for a short period of prewarming and then for warming therapy during anaesthesia. Additional infusion warming can be necessary if larger amounts of intravenous fluids are used. However, when a low flow rate is used, infusion warmers can be ineffective when standard tubing is used.

Transportation of newborns and preterm newborns from the neonatal intensive care unit to the operating room and back can be an important source of heat loss. In a prospective case control study, newborns that were operated on in the operating room were 10 times more likely to develop perioperative hypothermia compared to newborns that were operated on in the neonatal intensive care unit. Hypothermic children had more respiratory and cardio-circulatory problems after the operation [412]. Therefore surgery on preterm newborns in the neonatal intensive care unit should be preferred whenever possible.

Patients undergoing targeted temperature management
Unconscious survivors of out-of-hospital cardiac arrest have a high risk of poor neurologic function and therefore are treated with therapeutic hypothermia (32–34 °C) or targeted temperature management (36 °C) in the intensive care unit [413]. Sometimes patients need an operative intervention during this period. In this case the existing temperature management should be continued in the operating room, because massive changes in temperature [414] or the development of cerebral hyperthermia are associated with significantly poorer outcomes [415].

Chapter

34

Postoperative therapy

Most important adverse events that are associated with perioperative hypothermia develop in the postoperative period. However, only some of them, such as feeling cold and shivering [171] can be seen and treated in the direct postoperative phase. The more important consequences, such as morbid cardiac events [167] and surgical site infections [168], develop a few days later and to date no treatment can reverse these effects of perioperative hypothermia.

In the postanaesthetic care unit (PACU) some patients still arrive with hypothermia. In most of these patients optimal prevention of hypothermia was not accomplished or possible. Typical examples are:

- Emergency surgery where no time for prewarming was available
- Patients that arrived in the operating room with a low core temperature
- Patients with a high risk of perioperative hypothermia
- Operative procedures that were longer and more invasive than planned
- Operative procedures that could not be completed as planned, because of complications like massive bleeding.

Some of these patients may not be extubated when they are too cold and remain sedated until they are rewarmed again [129]. Therefore some hypothermic patients are admitted to the intensive care unit, which causes unnecessary costs [218]. There is no clear core temperature threshold below which patients should not be extubated, but many anaesthesiologists assume that patients should have a higher core temperature than 35.5 °C. We only know that a core temperature below 35 °C at admission to the PACU is associated with a higher risk of reintubation after planned extubation [181].

Additionally these patients may have:

- Postoperative thermal discomfort, which can be intense [171]
- Postoperative shivering [171]
- Significant bleeding due to the influence of hypothermia on the coagulation system [164]
- Prolonged action of muscle relaxants [142, 150].

As a consequence postanaesthetic recovery can be prolonged and these patients will have to stay longer in the PACU [178].

Therapeutic options

The therapeutic options in the PACU are active rewarming and treatment of shivering, if present.

Rewarming

Active rewarming aims mainly to speed up the rewarming, to reduce shivering and to increase thermal comfort.

Forced-air warming is the preferred method and is able to speed up rewarming [416, 417], reduce shivering [416] and to increase thermal comfort [418]. However, in some studies the rewarming process could not be accelerated [419], presumably because thermoregulatory vasoconstriction limited heat transfer from peripheral to central thermal compartments. As alternative measures, radiative warmers and conductive warmers have been used [357, 358].

Treatment of shivering

Postoperative shivering is common in hypothermic patients and is associated with thermal discomfort [418]. However, hypothermia is not the only reason for postanaesthetic shivering. It may also be caused by residual effects of volatile anaesthestics [173], remifentanil or pain [37, 174]. From a clinical point of view it can be difficult to differentiate between thermoregulatory shivering and non-thermoregulatory shivering. Typically patients with perioperative hypothermia and thermoregulatory shivering feel cold and have a lower postoperative core temperature compared with their individual preoperative value. They are almost always significantly vasoconstricted, which means that the temperature at the fingertips is lower than the temperature of the forearm [172].

Thermoregulatory shivering should be treated by active warming of the patient for two reasons:
1. It is the causal treatment
2. Active warming of the skin reduces the threshold for shivering by about 0.4 °C and thereby can sometimes stop shivering [418].

However, active warming alone very often is not sufficient to stop shivering and is not helpful against non-thermoregulatory shivering. In this case, additional treatment with drugs is advisable, although no treatment has ever been licensed for that purpose and the use of drugs to treat postoperative shivering is an off-label use of the drugs. Many substances have been shown to be effective against postoperative shivering:

- Meperidine [77, 420, 420–424]
- Alfentanil [421]
- Sufentanil [420]
- Nefopam [421, 425]
- Tramadol [78]

- Clonidine [73, 421, 423, 426–428]
- Dexmedetomidine [122, 427, 429]
- Urapidil [430]
- Ketanserin [428]
- Buspirone [424, 431]
- Ketamine [432]
- Doxapram [422]
- Physostigmin [423]
- Ondansetron [74, 433]
- Dolastetron and many more.

Meperidine and clonidine are very effective, with relatively few and well-known side effects [434]. The drugs should be titrated until shivering stops. Typical single doses for meperidine are 0.3 mg kg^{-1} and 2 µg kg^{-1} for clonidine. Alternative possibilities are tramadol or nefopam.

Patients should not leave the PACU until normothermia is achieved [20].

References

1. Von Hintzenstern U, Petermann H and Schwarz W. Frühe Erlanger Beiträge zur Theorie und Praxis der Äther- und Chloroformnarkose. Teil 2. Die tierexperimentellen Untersuchungen von Ernst von Bibra und Emil Harless. *Anaesthesist* 2001; **50**: 869–880.

2. Howland WS, Boyan CP and Schweizer O. Ventricular fibrillation during massive blood replacement. *Am J Surg* 1956; **92**: 356–360.

3. Boyan CP and Howland WS. Blood temperature: a critical factor in massive transfusion. *Anesthesiology* 1961; **22**: 559–563.

4. Churchill-Davidson HC. Some problems of massive blood transfusion. *Proc R Soc Med* 1968; **61**: 681–682.

5. France GG. Hypothermia in the newborn: body temperatures following anaesthesia. *Br J Anaesth* 1957; **29**: 390–396.

6. Hackett PR and Crosby RMN. Some effects of inadvertent hypothermia in infant neurosurgery. *Anesthesiology* 1960; **21**: 356–359.

7. Farman JV. Heat losses in infants undergoing surgery in air-conditioned theatres. *Br J Anaesth* 1962; **34**: 543–557.

8. Harrison GG, Bull AB and Schmidt HJ. Temperature changes in children during general anaesthesia. *Br J Anaesth* 1960; **32**: 60–68.

9. Boyan CP and Howland WS. Problems related to massive blood replacement. *Anesth Analg* 1962; **41**: 497–508.

10. Boyan CP and Howland WS. Cold or warmed blood for massive transfusions? *Anesth Analg* 1963; **42**: 142–146.

11. Bering EA, Jr. and Matson DD. A technic for the prevention of severe hypothermia during surgery of infants. *Ann Surg* 1953; **137**: 407–409.

12. Calvert DG. Inadvertent hypothermia in paediatric surgery and a method for its prevention. *Anaesthesia* 1962; **17**: 29–45.

13. Lewis RB, Shaw A and Etchells AH. Contact mattress to prevent heat loss in neonatal and paediatric surgery. *Br J Anaesth* 1973; **45**: 919–922.

14. Vaughan MS, Vaughan RW and Cork RC. Postoperative hypothermia in adults: relationship of age, anesthesia, and shivering to rewarming. *Anesth Analg* 1981; **60**: 746–751.

15. Roe CF, Goldberg MJ, Blair CS and Kinney JM. The influence of body temperature on early postoperative oxygen consumption. *Surgery* 1966; **60**: 85–92.

16. Sessler DI. The thermoregulation story. *Anesthesiology* 2013; **118**: 181–186.

17. NICE. Inadvertent perioperative hypothermia. The management of inadvertent perioperative hypothermia in adults. NICE Clinical Guideline 65. https://www.nice.org.uk/guidance/cg65/chapter/1-guidance, 2008.

18. Hooper VD, Chard R, Clifford T, *et al.* ASPAN's Evidence-Based Clinical Practice Guideline for the Promotion of Perioperative Normothermia: Second Edition. *J Perianesth Nurs* 2010; **25**: 346–365.

19. Forbes SS, Eskicioglu C, Nathens AB, *et al.* Evidence-based guidelines for prevention of perioperative hypothermia. *J Am Coll Surg* 2009; **209**: 492–503.

20. Torossian A, Bräuer A, Höcker J, *et al.* Preventing inadvertent perioperative hypothermia. *Dtsch Arztebl Int* 2015; **112**: 166–172.

21. Vriens J, Nilius B and Voets T. Peripheral thermosensation in mammals. *Nat Rev Neurosci* 2014; **15**: 573–589.

22. Schepers RJ and Ringkamp M. Thermoreceptors and thermosensitive afferents. *Neurosci Biobehav Rev* 2009; **33**: 205–212.

23. Craig AD. Interoception: the sense of the physiological condition of the body. *Curr Opin Neurobiol* 2003; **13**: 500–505.

24. Patapoutian A, Peier AM, Story GM and Viswanath V. ThermoTRP channels and beyond: mechanisms of temperature sensation. *Nat Rev Neurosci* 2003; **4**: 529–539.

25. Cauna N. The free penicillate nerve endings of the human hairy skin. *J Anat* 1973; **115**: 277–288.

26. Han ZS, Zhang ET and Craig AD. Nociceptive and thermoreceptive lamina I neurons are anatomically distinct. *Nat Neurosci* 1998; **1**: 218–225.

27. Craig AD. How do you feel? Interoception: the sense of the physiological condition of the body. *Nat Rev Neurosci* 2002; **3**: 655–666.

28. Blomqvist A, Zhang ET and Craig AD. Cytoarchitectonic and immunohistochemical characterization of a specific pain and temperature relay, the posterior portion of the ventral medial nucleus, in the human thalamus. *Brain* 2000; **123** Pt 3: 601–619.

29. Griffin JD, Saper CB and Boulant JA. Synaptic and morphological characteristics of temperature-sensitive and -insensitive rat hypothalamic neurones. *J Physiol* 2001; **537**: 521–535.

30. Flouris AD. Functional architecture of behavioural thermoregulation. *Eur J Appl Physiol* 2011; **111**: 1–8.

31. The Commission for Thermal Physiology of the International Union of Physiological Sciences. Glossary of Terms for Thermal Physiology: Third edition. *Jpn J Physiol* 2001; **51**: 245–280.

32. Sessler DI. Temperature monitoring and perioperative thermoregulation. *Anesthesiology* 2008; **109**: 318–338.

33. Bräuer A, Perl T and Quintel M. Perioperatives Wärmemanagement. *Anaesthesist* 2006; **55**: 1321–1340.

34. Romanovsky AA. Thermoregulation: some concepts have changed. Functional architecture of the thermoregulatory system. *Am J Physiol Regul Integr Comp Physiol* 2007; **292**: R37–R46.

35. Griffin JD and Boulant JA. Temperature effects on membrane potential and input resistance in rat hypothalamic neurones. *J Physiol* 1995; **488** Pt 2: 407–418.

36. Kushikata T, Hirota K, Kotani N, Yoshida H, Kudo M and Matsuki A. Isoflurane increases norepinephrine release in the rat preoptic area and the posterior hypothalamus in vivo and in vitro: relevance to thermoregulation during anesthesia. *Neuroscience* 2005; **131**: 79–86.

37. De Witte J and Sessler DI. Perioperative Shivering. *Anesthesiology* 2002; **96**: 467–484.

38. Frank SM, El-Gamal N, Raja SN, Wu PK and Afifi O. Role of alpha-adrenoceptors in the maintenance of core temperature in humans. *Clin Sci (Lond)* 1995; **89**: 219–225.

39. Kurz A, Sessler DI, Annadata R, *et al.* Midazolam minimally impairs thermoregulatory control. *Anesth Analg* 1995; **81**: 393–398.

40. Sessler DI, Olofsson CI, Rubinstein EH and Beebe JJ. The thermoregulatory threshold in humans during halothane anesthesia. *Anesthesiology* 1988; **68**: 836–842.

41. Sessler DI, Israel D, Pozos RS, Pozos M and Rubinstein EH. Spontaneous post-anesthetic tremor does not resemble thermoregulatory shivering. *Anesthesiology* 1988; **68**: 843–850.

42. Guffin A, Girard D and Kaplan JA. Shivering following cardiac surgery: hemodynamic changes and reversal. *J Cardiothorac Anesth* 1987; **1**: 24–28.

43. Sessler DI, Rubinstein EH and Moayeri A. Physiologic responses to mild perianesthetic hypothermia in humans. *Anesthesiology* 1991; **75**: 594–610.

44. Cannon B and Nedergaard J. Brown adipose tissue: function and physiological significance. *Physiol Rev* 2004; **84**: 277–359.

45. Plattner O, Semsroth M, Sessler DI, *et al.* Lack of nonshivering thermogenesis in infants anesthetized with fentanyl and propofol. *Anesthesiology* 1997; **86**: 772–777.

46. Weir JBdeV. New methods for calculating metabolic rate with special reference to protein metabolism. *J Physiol* 1949; **109**: 1–9.

47. Harris JA and Benedict FG. *A Biometric Study of Basal Metabolism in Man.* Washington DC: Lippicott Company, 1919.

48. English MJM. Physical principles of heat transfer. *Curr Anaesth Crit Care* 2001; **12**: 66–71.

49. English MJ and Hemmerling TM. Heat transfer coefficient: Medivance Arctic Sun Temperature Management System vs. water immersion. *Eur J Anaesthesiol* 2008; **25**: 531–537.

50. Bräuer A, Weyland W, Kazmaier S, *et al.* Efficacy of postoperative rewarming after cardiac surgery. *Ann Thorac Cardiovasc Surg* 2004; **10**: 171–177.

51. Kadam VR, Moyes D and Moran JL. Relative efficiency of two warming devices during laparoscopic cholecystectomy. *Anaesth Intensive Care* 2009; **37**: 464–468.

52. Bräuer A, Pacholik L, Perl T, *et al.* Conductive heat exchange with a gel-coated circulating water mattress. *Anesth Analg* 2004; **99**: 1742–1746.

53. Bräuer A, English MJM, Sander H, *et al.* Construction and evaluation of a manikin for perioperative heat exchange *Acta Anaesthesiol Scand* 2002; **46**: 43–50.

54. Hynson JM and Sessler DI. Intraoperative warming therapies: a comparison of three devices. *J Clin Anesth* 1992; **4**: 194–199.

55. Kurz A, Sessler DI, Christensen R and Dechert M. Heat balance and distribution during the core-temperature plateau in anesthetized humans. *Anesthesiology* 1995; **83**: 491–499.

56. Bickler PE and Sessler DI. Efficiency of airway heat and moisture exchangers in anesthetized humans. *Anesth Analg* 1990; **71**: 415–418.

57. Kurz A, Sessler DI, Narzt E, Lenhardt R and Lackner F. Morphometric influences on intraoperative core temperature changes. *Anesth Analg* 1995; **80**: 562–567.

58. Abelha FJ, Castro MA, Neves AM, Landeiro NM and Santos CC. Hypothermia in a surgical intensive care unit. *BMC Anesthesiology* 2005; **5**: 7–17.

59. Kongsayreepong S, Chaibundit C, Chadpaibool J, *et al.* Predictor of core hypothermia and the surgical intensive care unit. *Anesth Analg* 2003; **96**: 826–833.

60. Mehta OH and Barclay KL. Perioperative hypothermia in patients undergoing major colorectal surgery. *ANZ J Surg* 2014; **84**: 550–555.

61. Mitchell AM and Kennedy RR. Preoperative core temperatures in elective surgical patients show an unexpected skewed distribution. *Can J Anaesth* 2001; **48**: 850–853.

62. Frank SM, Kluger MJ and Kunkel SL. Elevated thermostatic setpoint in postoperative patients. *Anesthesiology* 2000; **93**: 1426–1431.

63. Torossian A, Bein B, Bräuer A, *et al.* S3 Leitlinie Vermeidung von perioperativer Hypothermie 2014. http://www.awmf.org/uploads/tx_szleitlinien/001-018l_S3_Vermeidung_perioperativer_Hypothermie_2014-05.pdf, 2014.

64. Bräuer A, Waeschle RM, Heise D, *et al.* Preoperative prewarming as a routine measure: first experiences. *Anaesthesist* 2010; **59**: 842–850.

65. Frank SM, Raja SN, Bulcao C and Goldstein DS. Age-related thermoregulatory differences during core cooling in humans. *Am J Physiol Regul Integr Comp Physiol* 2000; **279**: R349–R354.

66. Kurz A, Plattner O, Sessler DI, *et al.* The threshold for thermoregulatory vasoconstriction during nitrous oxide/isoflurane anesthesia is lower in elderly than in young patients. *Anesthesiology* 1993; **79**: 465–469.

67. Kitamura A, Hoshino T, Kon T and Ogawa R. Patients with diabetic neuropathy are at risk of a greater intraoperative reduction in core temperature. *Anesthesiology* 2000; **92**: 1311–1318.

68. Jonas JM, Ehrenkranz J and Gold MS. Urinary basal body temperature in anorexia nervosa. *Biol Psychiatry* 1989; **26**: 289–296.

69. Luck P and Wakeling A. Altered thresholds for thermoregulatory sweating and vasodilatation in anorexia nervosa. *Br Med J* 1980; **281**: 906–908.

70. Kudoh A, Takase H and Takazawa T. Chronic treatment with antidepressants decreases intraoperative core hypothermia. *Anesth Analg* 2003; **97**: 275–279.

71. Kudoh A, Takase H and Takazawa T. Chronic treatment with antipsychotics enhances intraoperative core hypothermia. *Anesth Analg* 2004; **98**: 111–115.

72. Matsukawa T, Hanagata K, Ozaki M, *et al.* I.m. midazolam as premedication produces a concentration-dependent decrease in core temperature in male volunteers. *Br J Anaesth* 1997; **78**: 396–399.

73. Nicolaou G, Chen AA, Johnston CE, *et al.* Clonidine decreases vasoconstriction and shivering thresholds, without affecting the sweating threshold. *Can J Anaesth* 1997; **44**: 636–642.

74. Powell RM and Buggy DJ. Ondansetron given before induction of anesthesia reduces shivering after general anesthesia. *Anesth Analg* 2000; **90**: 1423–1427.

75. Matsukawa T, Ozaki M, Nishiyama T, *et al.* Atropine prevents midazolam-induced core hypothermia in elderly patients. *J Clin Anesth* 2001; **13**: 504–508.

76. Kurz A, Go JC, Sessler DI, *et al.* Alfentanil slightly increases the sweating threshold and markedly reduces the vasoconstriction and shivering thresholds. *Anesthesiology* 1995; **83**: 293–299.

77. Kurz A, Ikeda T, Sessler DI, *et al.* Meperidine decreases the shivering threshold twice as much as the vasoconstriction threshold. *Anesthesiology* 1997; **86**: 1046–1054.

78. De Witte JL, Kim J-S, Sessler DI, Bastanmehr H and Bjorksten AR. Tramadol reduces the sweating, vasoconstriction, and shivering thresholds. *Anesth Analg* 1998; **87**: 173–179.

79. Sessler DI, Schroeder M, Merrifield B, Matsukawa T and Cheng C. Optimal duration and temperature of prewarming. *Anesthesiology* 1995; **82**: 674–681.

80. Matsukawa T, Sessler DI, Sessler AM, *et al.* Heat flow and distribution during induction of general anesthesia. *Anesthesiology* 1995; **82**: 662–673.

81. Matsukawa T, Sessler DI, Christensen R, Ozaki M and Schroeder M. Heat flow and distribution during epidural anesthesia. *Anesthesiology* 1995; **83**: 961–967.

82. Sessler DI. Complications and treatment of mild perioperative hypothermia. *Anesthesiology* 2001; **95**: 531–543.

83. Sessler DI. Mild perioperative hypothermia. *N Engl J Med* 1997; **336**: 1730–1737.

84. Matsukawa T, Kurz A, Sessler DI, *et al.* Propofol linearly reduces the vasoconstriction and shivering thresholds. *Anesthesiology* 1995; **82**: 1169–1180.

85. Washington DE, Sessler DI, McGuire J, *et al.* Painful stimulation minimally increases the thermoregulatory threshold for vasoconstriction during enflurane anesthesia in humans. *Anesthesiology* 1992; **77**: 286–290.

86. Xiong J, Kurz A, Sessler DI, *et al.* Isoflurane produces marked and nonlinear decreases in the vasoconstriction and shivering thresholds. *Anesthesiology* 1996; **85**: 240–245.

87. Ozaki M, Sessler DI, Suzuki H, *et al.* Nitrous oxide decreases the threshold for vasoconstriction less than sevoflurane or isoflurane. *Anesth Analg* 1995; **80**: 1212–1216.

88. Sessler DI, McGuire J, Hynson J, Moayeri A and Heier T. Thermoregulatory vasoconstriction during isoflurane anesthesia minimally decreases cutaneous heat loss. *Anesthesiology* 1992; **76**: 670–675.

89. Farber NE, Schmidt JE, Kampine JP and Schmeling WT. Halothane modulates thermosensitive hypothalamic neurons in rat brain slices. *Anesthesiology* 1995; **83**: 1241–1253.

90. El-Gamal N, El-Kassabany N, Frank SM, et al. Age-related thermoregulatory differences in a warm operating room environment (approximately 26°C). Anesth Analg 2000; **90**: 694–698.

91. Bissonnette B and Sessler DI. Thermoregulatory thresholds for vasoconstriction in pediatric patients anesthetized with halothane or halothane and caudal bupivacaine. Anesthesiology 1992; **76**: 387–392.

92. Joris J, Ozaki M, Sessler DI, et al. Epidural anesthesia impairs both central and peripheral thermoregulatory control during general anesthesia. Anesthesiology 1994; **80**: 268–277.

93. Smith D, Wood M, Pearson J, Mehta RL and Carli F. Effects of enflurane and isoflurane in air-oxygen on changes in thermal balance during and after surgery. Br J Anaesth 1990; **65**: 754–759.

94. Annadata R, Sessler DI, Tayefeh F, Kurz A and Dechert M. Desflurane slightly increases the sweating threshold but produces marked, nonlinear decreases in the vasoconstriction and shivering thresholds. Anesthesiology 1995; **83**: 1205–1211.

95. Sessler DI, Olofsson CI and Rubinstein EH. The thermoregulatory threshold in humans during nitrous oxide- fentanyl anesthesia. Anesthesiology 1988; **69**: 357–364.

96. An TH and Yang JW. Effects of PEEP on the thermoregulatory responses during TIVA in patients undergoing tympanoplasty. Korean J Anesthesiol 2011; **61**: 302–307.

97. Nakasuji M, Nakamura M, Imanaka N, et al. Intraoperative high-dose remifentanil increases post-anaesthetic shivering. Br J Anaesth 2010; **105**: 162–167.

98. Sessler DI. Perioperative heat balance. Anesthesiology 2000; **92**: 578–596.

99. Ikeda T, Kazama T, Sessler DI, et al. Induction of anesthesia with Ketamine reduces the magnitude of redistribution hypothermia. Anesth Analg 2001; **93**: 934–938.

100. Ikeda T, Sessler DI, Kitura M, et al. Less core hypothermia when anesthesia is induced with inhaled sevoflurane than with intravenous propofol. Anesth Analg 1999; **88**: 921–924.

101. Ikeda T, Ozaki M, Sessler DI, et al. Intraoperative phenylephrine infusion decreases the magnitude of redistribution hypothermia. Anesth Analg 1999; **89**: 462–465.

102. Horn EP, Bein B, Böhm R, et al. The effect of short time periods of pre-operative warming in the prevention of peri-operative hypothermia. Anaesthesia 2012; **67**: 612–617.

103. Perl T, Rhenius A, Eich C, et al. Conductive warming and insulation reduces perioperative hypothermia. Centr Eur J Med 2012; **7**: 284–289.

104. Witt L, Dennhardt N, Eich C, et al. Prevention of intraoperative hypothermia in neonates and infants: results of a prospective multicenter observational study with a new forced-air warming system with increased warm air flow. Paediatr Anaesth 2013; **23**: 469–474.

105. Sanders BJ, D'Alessio JG and Jernigan JR. Intraoperative hypothermia associated with lower extremity tourniquet deflation. J Clin Anesth 1996; **8**: 504–507.

106. Simon E. Thermoregulation as a switchboard of autonomic nervous and endocrine control. Jpn J Physiol 1999; **49**: 323.

107. Nakajima Y, Mizobe T, Matsukawa T, et al. Thermoregulatory response to intraoperative head-down tilt. Anesth Analg 2002; **94**: 221–226.

108. Nakajima Y, Mizobe T, Takamata A and Tanaka Y. Baroreflex modulation of peripheral vasoconstriction during progressive hypothermia in anesthetized humans. Am J Physiol Regul Integr Comp Physiol 2000; **279**: R1430–R1436.

109. Mizobe T, Nakajima Y, Sunaguchi M, Ueno H and Sessler DI. Clonidine produces a dose-dependent impairment of baroreflex-mediated thermoregulatory responses to positive end-expiratory

pressure in anaesthetized humans. *Br J Anaesth* 2005; **94**: 536–541.

110. Hynson JM, Sessler DI, Glosten B and McGuire J. Thermal balance and tremor patterns during epidural anesthesia. *Anesthesiology* 1991; **74**: 680–690.

111. Ozaki M, Kurz A, Sessler DI, *et al.* Thermoregulatory thresholds during epidural and spinal anesthesia. *Anesthesiology* 1994; **81**: 282–288.

112. Honarmand A and Safavi MR. Comparison of prophylactic use of midazolam, ketamine, and ketamine plus midazolam for prevention of shivering during regional anaesthesia: a randomized double-blind placebo controlled trial. *Br J Anaesth* 2008; **101**: 557–562.

113. Emerick TH, Ozaki M, Sessler DI, Walters K and Schroeder M. Epidural anesthesia increases apparent leg temperature and decreases the shivering threshold. *Anesthesiology* 1994; **81**: 289–298.

114. Kurz A, Sessler DI, Schroeder M and Kurz M. Thermoregulatory response thresholds during spinal anesthesia. *Anesth Analg* 1993; **77**: 721–726.

115. Frank SM, El-Rahmany HK, Cattaneo CG and Barnes RA. Predictors of hypothermia during spinal anesthesia. *Anesthesiology* 2000; **92**: 1330–1334.

116. Glosten B, Hynson J, Sessler DI and McGuire J. Preanesthetic skin-surface warming reduces redistribution hypothermia caused by epidural block. *Anesth Analg* 1993; **77**: 488–493.

117. Leslie K and Sessler DI. Reduction in the shivering threshold is proportional to spinal block height. *Anesthesiology* 1996; **84**: 1327–1331.

118. Frank SM, Shir Y, Raja SN, Fleisher LA and Beattie C. Core hypothermia and skin-surface temperature gradients: epidural versus general anesthesia and the effects of age. *Anesthesiology* 1994; **80**: 502–508.

119. Stjernström H, Henneberg S, Eklund A, *et al.* Thermal balance during transurethral resection of the prostate: a comparison of general anaesthesia and epidural analgesia. *Acta Anaesthesiol Scand* 1985; **29**: 743–749.

120. Szmuk P, Ezri T, Sessler DI, Stein A and Geva D. Spinal anesthesia speeds active postoperative rewarming. *Anesthesiology* 1997; **87**: 1050–1054.

121. Noguchi I, Matsukawa T, Ozaki M and Amemiya Y. Propofol in low doses causes redistribution of body heat in male volunteers. *Eur J Anaesthesiol* 2002; **19**: 677–681.

122. Talke P, Tayefeh F, Sessler DI, *et al.* Dexmedetomidine does not alter the sweating threshold, but comparably and linearly decreases the vasoconstriction and shivering thresholds. *Anesthesiology* 1997; **87**: 835–841.

123. Frank SM, Beattie C, Christopherson R, *et al.* Epidural versus general anesthesia, ambient operating room temperature, and patient age as predictors of inadvertent hypothermia. *Anesthesiology* 1992; **77**: 252–257.

124. von Dossow V, Welte M, Zaune U, *et al.* Thoracic epidural anesthesia combined with general anesthesia: the preferred anesthetic technique for thoracic surgery. *Anesth Analg* 2001; **92**: 848–854.

125. Heller AR, Litz RJ, Djonlagic I, *et al.* Combined anesthesia with epidural catheter: a retrospective analysis of the perioperative course in patients ungoing radical prostatectomy. *Anaesthesist* 2000; **49**: 949–959.

126. Pöpping DM, Elia N, Van Aken HK, *et al.* Impact of epidural analgesia on mortality and morbidity after surgery: systematic review and meta-analysis of randomized controlled trials. *Ann Surg* 2014; **259**: 1056–1067.

127. Long KC, Tanner EJ, Frey M, *et al.* Intraoperative hypothermia during primary surgical cytoreduction for advanced ovarian cancer: risk factors and associations with postoperative morbidity. *Gynecol Oncol* 2013; **131**: 525–530.

128. Bito H, Suzuki M and Shimada Y. Combination of thoracic epidural anesthesia does not always induce hypothermia during general anesthesia. *J Nippon Med Sch* 2008; **75**: 85–90.

129. Horn EP, Bein B, Broch O, *et al.* Warming before and after epidural block before general anaesthesia for major abdominal surgery prevents perioperative hypothermia: a randomised controlled trial. *Eur J Anaesthesiol* 2016; **33**: 334–340.

130. Clark RE, Orkin LR and Rovenstine EA. Body temperature studies in anesthetized man: effect of environmental temperature, humidity, and anesthesia system. *J Am Med Assoc* 1954; **154**: 311–319.

131. Morris RH and Kumar A. The effect of warming blankets on maintenance of body temperature of the anesthetized, paralysed patient. *Anesthesiology* 1972; **36**: 408–411.

132. Sessler DI, Sessler AM, Hudson S and Moayeri A. Heat loss during surgical skin preparation. *Anesthesiology* 1993; **78**: 1055–1064.

133. Lamke LO, Nilsson GE and Reither HL. Water loss by evaporation from the abdominal cavity during surgery. *Acta Chir Scand* 1977; **143**: 279–284.

134. Severens NM, Marken Lichtenbelt WD, Frijns AJ, *et al.* Temperature and surgical wound heat loss during orthopedic surgery: computer simulations and measurements. *Can J Anaesth* 2010; **57**: 381–382.

135. Pit MJ, Tegelaar RJ and Venema PL. Isothermic irrigation during transurethral resection of the prostate: effects on perioperative hypothermia, blood loss, resection time and patient satisfaction. *Br J Urol* 1996; **78**: 99–103.

136. Leijtens B, Koeter M, Kremers K and Koeter S. High incidence of postoperative hypothermia in total knee and total hip arthroplasty: a prospective observational study. *J Arthroplasty* 2013; **28**: 895–898.

137. Karalapillai D and Story D. Hypothermia on arrival in the intensive care unit after surgery. *Crit Care Resusc* 2008; **10**: 116–119.

138. Karalapillai D, Story DA, Calzavacca P, *et al.* Inadvertent hypothermia and mortality in postoperative intensive care patients: retrospective audit of 5050 patients. *Anaesthesia* 2009; **64**: 968–972.

139. Karalapillai D, Story D, Hart GK, *et al.* Postoperative hypothermia and patient outcomes after major elective non-cardiac surgery. *Anaesthesia* 2013; **68**: 605–611.

140. Sun Z, Honar H, Sessler DI, *et al.* Intraoperative core temperature patterns, transfusion requirement, and hospital duration in patients warmed with forced air. *Anesthesiology* 2015; **122**: 276–285.

141. Karalapillai D, Story D, Hart GK, *et al.* Postoperative hypothermia and patient outcomes after elective cardiac surgery. *Anaesthesia* 2011; **66**: 780–784.

142. Heier T, Caldwell JE, Sessler DI and Miller RD. Mild intraoperative hypothermia increases duration of action and spontaneous recovery of vecuronium blockade during nitrous oxide-isoflurane anesthesia in humans. *Anesthesiology* 1991; **74**: 815–819.

143. Heier T, Clough D, Wright PMC, *et al.* The influence of mild hypothermia on the pharmacokinetics and time course of action of Neostigmine in anesthetized volunteers. *Anesthesiology* 2002; **97**: 90–95.

144. Michelsen LG, Holford NH, Lu W, *et al.* The pharmacokinetics of remifentanil in patients undergoing coronary artery bypass grafting with cardiopulmonary bypass. *Anesth Analg* 2001; **93**: 1100–1105.

145. Bjelland TW, Klepstad P, Haugen BO, Nilsen T and Dale O. Effects of hypothermia on the disposition of morphine, midazolam, fentanyl, and propofol in intensive care unit patients. *Drug Metab Dispos* 2013; **41**: 214–223.

146. Zhou J and Poloyac SM. The effect of therapeutic hypothermia on drug metabolism and response: cellular mechanisms to organ function. *Expert Opin Drug Metab Toxicol* 2011; **7**: 803–816.

147. Zhou JX and Liu J. The effect of temperature on solubility of volatile anesthetics in human tissues. *Anesth Analg* 2001; **93**: 234–238.

148. Leslie K, Sessler DI, Bjorksten AR and Moayeri A. Mild hypothermia alters

propofol pharmacokinetics and increases the duration of action of atracurium. *Anesth Analg* 1995; **80**: 1007–1014.

149. Leslie K, Bjorksten AR, Ugoni A and Mitchell P. Mild core hypothermia and anesthetic requirement for loss of responsiveness during propofol anesthesia for craniotomy. *Anesth Analg* 2002; **94**: 1298–1303.

150. Beaufort AM, Wierda JM, Belopavlovic M, et al. The influence of hypothermia (surface cooling) on the time- course of action and on the pharmacokinetics of rocuronium in humans. *Eur J Anaesthesiol Suppl* 1995; **11**: 95–106.

151. Gruber M, Lindner R, Prasser C and Wiesner G. The effect of fluoride and hypothermia on the in vitro metabolism of Mivacurium. *Anesth Analg* 2002; **95**: 397–399.

152. Bachmann B, Biscoping J, Sinnig E and Hempelmann G. Protein binding of prilocain in human plasma: influence of concentration, pH and temperature. *Acta Anaesthesiol Scand* 1990; **34**: 311–314.

153. Rajagopalan S, Mascha E and Sessler DI. The effects of mild perioperative hypothermia on blood loss and transfusion requirement. *Anesthesiology* 2008; **108**: 71–77.

154. Hewlett L, Zupancic G, Mashanov G, et al. Temperature-dependence of Weibel–Palade body exocytosis and cell surface dispersal of von Willebrand factor and its propolypeptide. *PLoS One* 2011; **6**: e27314.

155. Wolberg AS, Meng ZH, Monroe DM III and Hoffman M. A systematic evaluation of the effect of temperature on coagulation enzyme activity and platelet function. *J Trauma* 2004; **56**: 1221–1228.

156. Valeri CR, MacGregor H, Cassidy G, Tinney R and Pompei F. Effects of temperature on bleeding time and clotting time in normal male and female volunteers. *Crit Care Med* 1995; **23**: 698–704.

157. Rohrer MJ and Natale AM. Effect of hypothermia on the coagulation cascade. *Crit Care Med* 1992; **20**: 1402–1405.

158. Dirkmann D, Hanke AA, Görlinger K and Peters J. Hypothermia and acidosis synergistically impair coagulation in human whole blood. *Anesth Analg* 2008; **106**: 1627–1632.

159. Frey JM, Svegby HK, Svenarud PK and van der Linden JA. CO2 insufflation influences the temperature of the open surgical wound. *Wound Repair Regen* 2010; **18**: 378–382.

160. English MJ, Papenberg R, Farias E, Scott WA and Hinchey J. Heat loss in an animal experimental model. *J Trauma* 1991; **31**: 36–38.

161. Frey JM, Janson M, Svanfeldt M, Svenarud PK and van der Linden JA. Local Insufflation of warm humidified CO_2 increases open wound and core temperature during open colon surgery: a randomized clinical trial. *Anesth Analg* 2012; **115**: 1204–1211.

162. Just B, Trevien V, Delva E and Lienhart A. Prevention of intraoperative hypothermia by preoperative skin-surface warming. *Anesthesiology* 1993; **79**: 214–218.

163. Bräuer A, Perl T, Wittkopp E, Braun U and Weyland W. Stellenwert eines reflektierenden Isolationsmaterials (Thermadrape) zur Verhinderung intraoperativer Hypothermie. *Anaesthesiol Intensivmed Notfallmed Schmerzther* 2000; **35**: 756–762.

164. Schmied H, Kurz A, Sessler DI, Kozek S and Reiter A. Mild hypothermia increases blood loss and transfusion requirements during total hip arthroplasty. *Lancet* 1996; **347**: 289–292.

165. Hofer CK, Worn M, Tavakoli R, et al. Influence of body core temperature on blood loss and transfusion requirements during off-pump coronary artery bypass grafting: a comparison of 3 warming systems. *J Thorac Cardiovasc Surg* 2005; **129**: 838–843.

166. Bock M, Müller J, Bach A, et al. Effects of preinduction and intraoperative warming during major laparotomy. *Br J Anaesth* 1998; **80**: 159–163.

167. Frank SM, Fleisher LA, Breslow MJ, et al. Perioperative maintenance of

normothermia reduces the incidence of morbid cardiac events: a randomized clinical trial. *JAMA* 1997; **277**: 1127–1134.

168. Kurz A, Sessler DI and Lenhardt R. Study of Wound Infection and Temperature Group. Perioperative normothermia to reduce the incidence of surgical-wound infection and shorten hospitalization. *N Engl J Med* 1996; **334**: 1209–1215.

169. Moslemi-Kebria M, El-Nashar SA, Aletti GD and Cliby WA. Intraoperative hypothermia during cytoreductive surgery for ovarian cancer and perioperative morbidity. *Obstet Gynecol* 2012; **119**: 590–596.

170. Schmied H, Schiferer A, Sessler DI and Meznik C. The effects of red-cell scavenging, hemodilution, and active warming on allogenic blood requirements in patients undergoing hip or knee arthroplasty. *Anesth Analg* 1998; **86**: 387–391.

171. Kurz A, Sessler DI, Narzt E, *et al.* Postoperative hemodynamic and thermoregulatory consequences of intraoperative core hypothermia. *J Clin Anesth* 1995; **7**: 359–366.

172. Horn EP. Postoperative shivering: aetiology and treatment. *Curr Opin Anaesthesiol* 1999; **12**: 449–453.

173. Horn E-P, Sessler DI, Standl T, *et al.* Non-thermoregulatory shivering in patients recovering from Isoflurane or Desflurane anesthesia. *Anesthesiology* 1998; **88**: 878–886.

174. Horn EP, Schroeder F, Wilhelm S, *et al.* Postoperative pain facilitates nonthermoregulatory tremor. *Anesthesiology* 1999; **91**: 979–984.

175. Frank SM, Fleisher LA, Olson KF, *et al.* Multivariate determinants of early postoperative oxygen consumption in elderly patients: effects of shivering, body temperature, and gender. *Anesthesiology* 1995; **83**: 241–249.

176. Frank SM, Beattie C, Christopherson R, *et al.* The Perioperative Ischemia Randomized Anesthesia Trial Study Group. Unintentional hypothermia is associated with postoperative myocardial

ischemia. *Anesthesiology* 1993; **78**: 468–476.

177. Sladen RN. Thermal regulation in anesthesia and surgery. In Barash PG (ed.), *ASA Refresher Course*. Philadelphia: J.B. Lippincott Company, 1991: 165–187.

178. Lenhardt R, Marker E, Goll V, *et al.* Mild intraoperative hypothermia prolongs postanesthetic recovery. *Anesthesiology* 1997; **87**: 1318–1323.

179. Frank SM, Higgins MS, Breslow MJ, *et al.* The catecholamine, cortisol, and hemodynamic responses to mild perioperative hypothermia: a randomized clinical trial. *Anesthesiology* 1995; **82**: 83–93.

180. Smith CE, Gerdes E, Sweda S, *et al.* Warming intravenous fluids reduces perioperative hypothermia in women undergoing ambulatory gynecological surgery. *Anesth Analg* 1998; **87**: 37–41.

181. Lin HT, Ting PC, Chang WY, *et al.* Predictive risk index and prognosis of postoperative reintubation after planned extubation during general anesthesia: a single-center retrospective case-controlled study in Taiwan from 2005 to 2009. *Acta Anaesthesiol Taiwan* 2013; **51**: 3–9.

182. Bissonnette B, Sessler DI and LaFlamme P. Passive and active inspired gas humidification in infants and children. *Anesthesiology* 1989; **71**: 350–354.

183. Pagnocca ML, Tai EJ and Dwan JL. Temperature control in conventional abdominal surgery: comparison between conductive and the association of conductive and convective warming. *Rev Bras Anestesiol* 2009; **59**: 61.

184. Goldstein DS and Frank SM. The wisdom of the body revisited: the adrenomedullary response to mild core hypothermia in humans. *Endocr Regul* 2001; **35**: 3–7.

185. Frank SM, Cattaneo CG, Wieneke-Brady MB, *et al.* Threshold for adrenomedullary activation and increased cardiac work during mild core hypothermia. *Clin Sci (Lond)* 2002; **102**: 119–125.

186. Frank SM, Satitpunwaycha P, Bruce SR, Herscovitch P and Goldstein DS. Increased myocardial perfusion and

sympathoadrenal activation during mild core hypothermia in awake humans. *Clin Sci (Lond)* 2003; **104**: 503–508.

187. Billeter AT, Hohmann SF, Druen D, Cannon R and Polk HC, Jr. Unintentional perioperative hypothermia is associated with severe complications and high mortality in elective operations. *Surgery* 2014; **156**: 1245–1252.

188. Scott AV, Stonemetz JL, Wasey JO, *et al.* Compliance with Surgical Care Improvement Project for Body Temperature Management (SCIP Inf-10) is associated with improved clinical outcomes. *Anesthesiology* 2015; **123**: 116–125.

189. Landesberg G, Beattie WS, Mosseri M, Jaffe AS and Alpert JS. Perioperative myocardial infarction. *Circulation* 2009; **119**: 2936–2944.

190. Fleisher LA, Beckman JA, Brown KA, *et al.* ACC/AHA 2007 Guidelines on Perioperative Cardiovascular Evaluation and Care for Noncardiac Surgery. Executive summary: a report of the American College of Cardiology/ American Heart Association Task Force on Practice Guidelines (Writing Committee to Revise the 2002 Guidelines on Perioperative Cardiovascular Evaluation for Noncardiac Surgery) developed in collaboration with the American Society of Echocardiography, American Society of Nuclear Cardiology, Heart Rhythm Society, Society of Cardiovascular Anesthesiologists, Society for Cardiovascular Angiography and Interventions, Society for Vascular Medicine and Biology, and Society for Vascular Surgery. *J Am Coll Cardiol* 2007; **50**: 1707–1732.

191. Mauermann WJ and Nemergut EC. The anesthesiologist's role in the prevention of surgical site infections. *Anesthesiology* 2006; **105**: 413–421.

192. Melling AC, Ali B, Scott EM and Leaper DJ. Effects of preoperative warming on the incidence of wound infection after clean surgery: a randomised controlled trial. *Lancet* 2001; **358**: 876–880.

193. Sessler DI. Non-pharmacologic prevention of surgical wound infection. *Anesthesiol Clin* 2006; **24**: 279–297.

194. Sheffield CW, Sessler DI, Hopf HW, *et al.* Centrally and locally mediated thermoregulatory responses alter subcutaneous oxygen tension. *Wound Rep Reg* 1996; **4**: 339–345.

195. Hopf HW, Hunt TK, West JM, *et al.* Wound tissue oxygen tension predicts the risk of wound infection in surgical patients. *Arch Surg* 1997; **132**: 997–1004.

196. Van Oss CM, Absolom DR, Moore LL, Park BH and Humbert JR. Effect of temperature on the chemotaxis, phagocytotic engulfment, digestion and O2 consumption of human polynuclear leukocytes. *J Reticuloendothelial Soc* 1980; **27**: 561–565.

197. Wenisch C, Narzt E, Sessler DI, *et al.* Mild intraoperative hypothermia reduces production of reactive oxygen intermediates by polymorphonuclear leukocytes. *Anesth Analg* 1996; **82**: 810–816.

198. Beilin B, Shavit Y, Razumovsky J, *et al.* Effects of mild perioperative hypothermia on cellular immune responses. *Anesthesiology* 1998; **89**: 1133–1140.

199. Qadan M, Gardner SA, Vitale DS, *et al.* Hypothermia and surgery: immunologic mechanisms for current practice. *Ann Surg* 2009; **250**: 134–140.

200. Barone JE, Tucker JB, Cecere J, *et al.* Hypothermia does not result in more complications after colon surgery. *Am Surg* 1999; **65**: 356–359.

201. Melling AC and Leaper DJ. The impact of warming on pain and wound healing after hernia surgery: a preliminary study. *J Wound Care* 2006; **15**: 104–108.

202. Shabino PJ, Khoraki J, Elegbede AF, *et al.* Reduction of surgical site infections after laparoscopic gastric bypass with circular stapled gastrojejunostomy. *Surg Obes Relat Dis* 2016; **12**: 4–9.

203. Flores-Maldonado A, Medina-Escobedo CE, Rios-Rodriguez HMG and Fernandez-

Dominguez R. Mild perioperative hypothermia and the risk of wound infection. *Arch Med Res* 2001; **32**: 227–231.

204. Seamon MJ, Wobb J, Gaughan JP, *et al.* The effects of intraoperative hypothermia on surgical site infection: an analysis of 524 trauma laparotomies. *Ann Surg* 2012; **255**: 789–795.

205. Hill JB, Sexton KW, Bartlett EL, *et al.* The clinical role of intraoperative core temperature in free tissue transfer. *Ann Plast Surg* 2015; **75**: 620–624.

206. Agrawal N, Sewell DA, Griswold ME, *et al.* Hypothermia during head and neck surgery. *Laryngoscope* 2003; **113**: 1278–1282.

207. Melton GB, Vogel JD, Swenson BR, *et al.* Continuous intraoperative temperature measurement and surgical site infection risk: analysis of anesthesia information system data in 1008 colorectal procedures. *Ann Surg* 2013; **258**: 606–612.

208. Gerszten PC, Albright AL, Pollack IF and Adelson PD. Intraoperative hypothermia and ventricular shunt infections. *Acta Neurochir (Wien)* 1998; **140**: 591–594.

209. Leijtens B, Koeter M, Kremers K and Koeter S. High incidence of postoperative hypothermia in total knee and total hip arthroplasty: a prospective observational study. *J Arthroplasty* 2013; **28**: 895–898.

210. Linam WM, Margolis PA, Staat MA, *et al.* Risk factors associated with surgical site infection after pediatric posterior spinal fusion procedure. *Infect Control Hosp Epidemiol* 2009; **30**: 109–116.

211. Edwards RK, Madani K and Duff P. Is perioperative hypothermia a risk factor for post-cesarean infection? *Infect Dis Obstet Gynecol* 2003; **11**: 75–80.

212. Carli F, Clark MM and Woollen JW. Investigation of the relationship between heat loss and nitrogen excretion in elderly patients undergoing major abdominal surgery under general anaesthetic. *Br J Anaesth* 1982; **54**: 1023–1029.

213. Carli F and Itiaba K. Effect of heat conservation during and after major abdominal surgery on muscle protein breakdown in elderly patients. *Br J Anaesth* 1986; **58**: 502–507.

214. Carli F, Emery PW and Freemantle CA. Effect of peroperative normothermia on postoperative protein metabolism in elderly patients undergoing hip arthroplasty. *Br J Anaesth* 1989; **63**: 276–282.

215. Carli F, Gabrielczyk M, Clark MM and Aber VR. An investigation of factors affecting postoperative rewarming of adult patients. *Anaesthesia* 1986; **41**: 363–369.

216. Yücel Y, Barlan M, Lenhardt R, Kurz A and Sessler DI. Perioperative hypothermia does not enhance the risk of cancer dissemination. *Am J Surg* 2005; **189**: 651–655.

217. Ben-Eliyahu S, Shakhar G, Rosenne E, Levinson Y and Beilin B. Hypothermia in barbiturate-anesthetized rats suppresses natural killer cell activity and compromises resistance to tumor metastasis: a role for adrenergic mechanisms. *Anesthesiology* 1999; **91**: 732–740.

218. Bauer M, Bock M, Martin J *et al.* Ungeplante postoperative Aufnahme elektiver Patienten auf Intensivstation: Eine prospektive Multi-Center-Analyse von Inzidenz, Kausalität und Vermeidbarkeit. *Anästh Intensivmed* 2007; **48**: 542–550.

219. Bush HL, Jr., Hydo LJ, Fischer E, *et al.* Hypothermia during elective abdominal aortic aneurysm repair: the high price of avoidable morbidity. *J Vasc Surg* 1995; **21**: 392–400.

220. Quiroga E, Tran NT, Hatsukami T and Starnes BW. Hypothermia is associated with increased mortality in patients undergoing repair of ruptured abdominal aortic aneurysm. *J Endovasc Ther* 2010; **17**: 434–438.

221. Janczyk RJ, Howells GA, Bair HA, *et al.* Hypothermia is an independent predictor of mortality in ruptured abdominal aortic aneurysms. *Vasc Endovascular Surg* 2004; **38**: 37–42.

222. Fecho K, Lunney AT, Boysen PG, Rock P and Norfleet EA. Postoperative mortality after inpatient surgery: incidence and risk factors. *Ther Clin Risk Manag* 2008; **4**: 681–688.

223. Crawford DC, Hicks B and Thompson MJ. Which thermometer? Factors influencing best choice for intermittent clinical temperature assessment. *J Med Eng Technol* 2006; **30**: 199–211.

224. Clark RP and Edholm OG. *Man and His Thermal Environment*. London: Edward Arnold Publishers Ltd, 1985.

225. Brandes IF, Perl T, Bauer M and Bräuer A. Evaluation of a novel noninvasive continuous core temperature measurement system with a zero heat flux sensor using a manikin of the human body. *Biomed Tech (Berl)* 2015; **60**: 1–9.

226. Eshraghi Y, Nasr V, Parra-Sanchez I, *et al.* An evaluation of a zero-heat-flux cutaneous thermometer in cardiac surgical patients. *Anesth Analg* 2014; **119**: 543–549.

227. Iden T, Horn EP, Bein B, *et al.* Intraoperative temperature monitoring with zero heat flux technology (3M SpotOn sensor) in comparison with sublingual and nasopharyngeal temperature: an observational study. *Eur J Anaesthesiol* 2015; **32**: 387–391.

228. Kimberger O, Thell R, Schuh M, *et al.* Accuracy and precision of a novel non-invasive core thermometer. *Br J Anaesth* 2009; **103**: 226–231.

229. Kimberger O, Saager L, Egan C, *et al.* The accuracy of a disposable noninvasive core thermometer. *Can J Anaesth* 2013; **60**: 1190–1196.

230. Wartzek T, Mühlsteff J and Imhoff M. Temperature measurement. *Biomed Tech (Berl)* 2011; **56**: 241–257.

231. Whitby JD and Dunkin LJ. Temperature differences in the oesophagus: the effects of intubation and ventilation. *Br J Anaesth* 1969; **41**: 615–618.

232. Mekjavic IB and Rempel ME. Determination of esophageal probe insertion length based on standing and sitting height. *J Appl Physiol* 1990; **69**: 376–379.

233. Whitby JD and Dunkin LJ. Oesophageal temperature differences in children. *Br J Anaesth* 1970; **42**: 1013–1015.

234. Alvord LS and Farmer BL. Anatomy and orientation of the human external ear. *J Am Acad Audiol* 1997; **8**: 383–390.

235. Lopez M, Sessler DI, Walter K, Emerick T and Ozaki M. Rate and gender dependence of the sweating, vasoconstriction, and shivering thresholds in humans. *Anesthesiology* 1994; **80**: 780–788.

236. Schuhmann MU, Suhr DF, v.Gösseln HH *et al.* Local brain surface temperature compared to temperatures measured at standard extracranial monitoring sites during posterior fossa surgery. *J Neurosurg Anesthesiol* 1999; **11**: 90–95.

237. Wallace CT, Marks WE, Adskins WY and Mahaffey JE. Perforation of the tympanic membrane, a complication of tympanic thermometry during anesthesia. *Anesthesiology* 1974; **41**: 290–291.

238. Lefrant J-Y, Muller L, Emmanuel Coussaye J, *et al.* Temperature measurement in intensive care patients: comparison of urinary bladder, oesophageal, rectal, axillary, and inguinal methods versus pulmonary artery core method. *Intensive Care Med* 2003; **29**: 414–418.

239. Torossian A. Survey on intraoperative temperature management in Europe. *Eur J Anaesthesiol* 2007; **24**: 668–675.

240. Bräuer A, Russo M, Nickel EA, Bauer M and Russo SG. Anwendungsrealität des perioperativen Wärmemanagements in Deutschland. Ergebnisse einer Online-Umfrage. *Anästh Intensivmed* 2015; **56**: 287–297.

241. Lee J, Lim H, Son KG and Ko S. Optimal nasopharyngeal temperature probe placement. *Anesth Analg* 2014; **119**: 875–879.

242. Knapik P, Rychlik W, Duda D, *et al.* Relationship between blood, nasopharyngeal and urinary bladder temperature during intravascular cooling for therapeutic hypothermia after cardiac arrest. *Resuscitation* 2012; **83**: 208–212.

243. Snoek AP and Saffer E. Agreement between lower esophageal and

nasopharyngeal temperatures in children ventilated with an endotracheal tube with leak. *Paediatr Anaesth* 2016; **26**: 213–220.

244. Wang M, Singh A, Qureshi H, *et al.* Optimal depth for nasopharyngeal temperature probe positioning. *Anesth Analg* 2016; **122**: 1434–1438.

245. Höcker J, Bein B, Böhm R, *et al.* Correlation, accuracy, precision and practicability of perioperative measurement of sublingual temperature in comparison with tympanic membrane temperature in awake and anaesthetised patients. *Eur J Anaesthesiol* 2012; **29**: 70–74.

246. Bräuer A, Weyland W, Fritz U, *et al.* Bestimmung der Körperkerntemperatur. Ein Vergleich von Ösophagus-, Blasen- und Rektaltemperatur während der postoperativen Wiedererwärmung. *Anaesthesist* 1997; **46**: 683–688.

247. Nierman DM. Core temperature measurement in the intensive care unit. *Crit Care Med* 1991; **19**: 818–823.

248. Bräuer A, Martin J-D, Schuhmann MU, Braun U and Weyland W. Genauigkeit der Blasentemperaturmessung bei intraabdominellen Eingriffen. *Anaesthesiol Intensivmed Notfallmed Schmerzther* 2000; **35**: 435–439.

249. Sato H, Yamakage M, Okuyama K, *et al.* Urinary bladder and oesophageal temperatures correlate better in patients with high rather than low urinary flow rates during non-cardiac surgery. *Eur J Anaesthesiol* 2008; **25**: 805–809.

250. Bissonnette B, Sessler DI and LaFlamme P. Intraoperative temperature monitoring sites in infants and children and the effect of inspired gas warming on esophageal temperature. *Anesth Analg* 1989; **69**: 192–196.

251. Fritz U, Rohrberg M, Lange C, *et al.* Infrarot-Temperaturmessung in Gehörgang mit dem DIATEK 9000 Instatemp und dem DIATEK 9000 Thermoguide: Einflussgrössen und Vergleich mit anderen Methoden der Temperaturmessung des Körperkerns. *Anaesthesist* 1996; **45**: 1059–1066.

252. Rohrberg M, Fritz U, Weyland W and Braun U. Temperaturmessung in Gehörgang: Vergleich eines Infrarot-Thermometers mit konventionellen Temperatursonden und Evaluation klinischer Einflugrössen auf die Infrarot-Messung. *Anaesthesiol Intensivmed Notfallmed Schmerzther* 1997; **32**: 403–412.

253. Kimberger O, Cohen D, Illevich U and Lenhardt R. Temporal artery versus bladder thermometry during perioperative and intensive care unit monitoring. *Anesth Analg* 2007; **105**: 1042–1047.

254. Bräuer A, Bovenschulte H, Perl T, *et al.* What determines the efficacy of forced-air warming systems?: a manikin evaluation with upper body blankets. *Anesth Analg* 2009; **108**: 192–198.

255. Kurz A, Kurz M, Poeschl G, *et al.* Forced-air warming maintains intraoperative normothermia better than circulating-water mattresses. *Anesth Analg* 1993; **77**: 89–95.

256. Vanni SM, Braz JR, Módolo NS, Amorin RB and Rodrigues GRJ. Preoperative combined with intraoperative skin-surface warming avoids hypothermia caused by general anesthesia and surgery. *J Clin Anesth* 2007; **15**: 119–125.

257. Vanni SMD, Castiglia YMM, Ganem EM, *et al.* Preoperative warming combined with intraoperative skin-surface warming does not avoid hypothermia cuased by spinal anesthesia in patients with midazolam premedication. *Sao Paulo Med J* 2007; **125**: 144–149.

258. Andrzejowski J, Hoyle J, Eapen G and Turnbull D. Effect of prewarming on post-induction core temperature and the incidence of inadvertent perioperative hypothermia in patients undergoing general anaesthesia. *Br J Anaesth* 2008; **101**: 627–631.

259. Perl T, Peichl LH, Reyntjens K, *et al.* Efficacy of a novel prewarming system in the prevention of perioperative hypothermia: a prospective, randomized, multicenter study. *Minerva Anestesiol* 2014; **80**: 436–443.

260. Bräuer A and Quintel M. Forced-air warming: technology, physical background and practical aspects. *Curr Opin Anaesthesiol* 2009; **22**: 769–774.

261. Bräuer A, English MJM, Steinmetz N, et al. Efficacy of forced-air warming systems with full body blankets. [Efficacite des systemes de chauffage a air pulse avec des couvertures a champ complet]. *Can J Anaesth* 2007; **54**: 34–41.

262. Bräuer A, English MJM, Steinmetz N, et al. Comparison of forced-air warming systems with upper body blankets using a copper manikin of the human body. *Acta Anaesthesiol Scand* 2002; **46**: 965–972.

263. Bräuer A, English MJM, Sander H, et al. Construction and evaluation of a manikin for perioperative heat exchange. *Acta Anaesthesiol Scand* 2002; **46**: 43–50.

264. Perl T, Bräuer A, Timmermann A, Braun U and Weyland W. Differences among forced-air warming systems with upper body blankets are small: a randomized trial for heat transfer in volunteers. *Acta Anaesthesiol Scand* 2003; **47**: 1159–1164.

265. Bräuer A, English MJ, Lorenz N, et al. Comparison of forced-air warming systems with lower body blankets using a copper manikin of the human body. *Acta Anaesthesiol Scand* 2003; **47**: 58–64.

266. Wagner K, Swanson E, Raymond CJ and Smith CE. Comparison of two convective warming systems during major abdominal and orthopedic surgery. *Can J Anesth* 2008; **55**: 358–363.

267. Camus Y, Delva E, Just B and Lienhart A. Leg warming minimizes core hypothermia during abdominal surgery. *Anesth Analg* 1993; **77**: 995–999.

268. Bräuer A and Quintel M. Comprendre la technologie et les principes physiques des matelas à air pulsé. *Le Praticien en Anesthésie Réanimation* 2011; **15**: 281–286.

269. Leben J and Tryba M. Prevention of hypothermia during surgery: contribuation of convective heating system and warm infusion. *Ann N Y Acad Sci* 1997; **813**: 807–811.

270. Ihn CH, Joo JD, Chung HS, et al. Comparison of three warming devices for the prevention of core hypothermia and post-anaesthesia shivering. *J Int Med Res* 2008; **36**: 923–931.

271. Motamed C, Labaille T, Leon O, et al. Core and thenar skin temperature variation during prolonged abdominal surgery: comparison of two sites of active forced air warming. *Acta Anaesthesiol Scand* 2000; **44**: 249–254.

272. Triffterer L, Marhofer P, Sulyok I, et al. Forced-air warming during pediatric surgery: a randomized comparison of a compressible with a noncompressible warming system. *Anesth Analg* 2016; **122**: 219–225.

273. Uzun G, Mutluoglu M, Evinc R, Ozdemir Y and Sen H. Severe burn injury associated with misuse of forced-air warming device. *J Anesth* 2010; **24**: 980–981.

274. Azzam FJ and Krock JL. Thermal burns in two infants associated with a forced air warming system [letter]. *Anesth Analg* 1995; **81**: 661.

275. Mehta S. Burn injuries from warming devices in the operating room. *ASA Monitor* 2013; **77**: 16–17.

276. English MJ, Farmer C and Scott WA. Heat loss in exposed volunteers. *J Trauma* 1990; **30**: 422–425.

277. Golden S and Bachmann C. Forced air warmer burn can occur with poor circulation. *APSF Newsletter* 2006; **20**: 87.

278. Eich C, Zink W, Schwarz SKW, Radke O and Bräuer A. A combination of convective and conductive warming ensures pre- and post-bypass normothermia in paediatric cardiac anaesthesia. *Appl Cardiopulmon Pathophysiol* 2009; **13**: 3–10.

279. Stewart C and Harban F. Thermal injuries from the use of a forced-air warming device. *Paediatr Anaesth* 2012; **22**: 414–415.

280. Pham AK and Ravanfar P. Distinctive cutaneous findings due to a rare complication from a warming device. *J Am Acad Dermatol* 2014; **71**: e76–e77.

281. Siddik-Sayyid SM, Saasouh WA, Mallat CE and Aouad MT. Thermal burn following combined use of forced air and fluid warming devices. *Anaesthesia* 2010; **65**: 654–655.

282. Bräuer A, Perl T, Heise D, Quintel M and Seipelt R. Intraoperative full-thickness pressure ulcer in a patient after transapical aortic valve replacement using a novel underbody forced-air warming blanket. *J Clin Anesth* 2010; **22**: 573–574.

283. Scott EM, Leaper DJ, Clark M and Kelly PJ. Effects of warming therapy on pressure ulcers: a randomized trial. *AORN J* 2001; **73**: 921–33, 936.

284. Albrecht M, Gauthier RL, Belani K, Litchy M and Leaper D. Forced-air warming blowers: an evaluation of filtration adequacy and airborne contamination emissions in the operating room. *Am J Infect Control* 2011; **39**: 321–328.

285. Avidan MS, Jones N, Ing R, *et al.* Convection warmers: not just hot air. *Anaesthesia* 1997; **52**: 1073–1076.

286. Baker N, King D and Smith EG. Infection control hazards of intraoperative forced air warming. *J Hosp Infect* 2002; **51**: 153–154.

287. Bernards AT, Harinck HI, Dijkshoorn L, van der Reijden TJ and van den Broek PJ. Persistent *Acinetobacter baumannii*? Look inside your medical equipment. *Infect Control Hosp Epidemiol* 2004; **25**: 1002–1004.

288. Zink RS and Iaizzo PA. Convective warming therapy does not increase the risk of wound contamination in the operating room. *Anesth Analg* 1993; **76**: 50–53.

289. Sharp RJ, Chesworth T and Fern ED. Do warming blankets increase bacterial counts in the operating field in a laminar-flow theatre? *J Bone Joint Surg (Br)* 2002; **84 B**: 486–488.

290. Moretti B, Larocca AM, Napoli C, *et al.* Active warming systems to maintain perioperative normothermia in hip replacement surgery: a therapeutic aid or a vector of infection? *J Hosp Infect* 2009; **73**: 58–63.

291. McGovern PD, Albrecht M, Belani KG, *et al.* Forced-air warming and ultra-clean ventilation do not mix: an investigation of theatre ventilation, patient warming and joint replacement infection in orthopaedics. *J Bone Joint Surg Br* 2011; **93**: 1537–1544.

292. Thiele RH, Huffmyer JL and Nemergut EC. The 'six sigma approach' to the operating room environment and infection. *Best Pract Res Clin Anaesthesiol* 2008; **22**: 537–552.

293. Yang L, Huang CY, Zhou ZB, *et al.* Risk factors for hypothermia in patients under general anesthesia: Is there a drawback of laminar airflow operating rooms?: a prospective cohort study. *Int J Surg* 2015; **21**: 14–17.

294. Dasari KB, Albrecht M and Harper M. Effect of forced-air warming on the performance of operating theatre laminar flow ventilation. *Anaesthesia* 2012; **67**: 244–249.

295. Belani KG, Albrecht M, McGovern PD, Reed M and Nachtsheim C. Patient warming excess heat: the effects on orthopedic operating room ventilation performance. *Anesth Analg* 2013; **117**: 406–411.

296. Sessler DI, Olmsted RN and Kuelpmann R. Forced-air warming does not worsen air quality in laminar flow operating rooms. *Anesth Analg* 2011; **113**: 1416–1421.

297. Austin PN. The information age and hot air. *AANA J* 2015; **83**: 237–239.

298. [No authors listed] Forced-air warming and surgical site infections. Our review finds insufficient evidence to support changes in current practice. *Health Devices* 2013; **42**: 122–125.

299. Brandt S, Oguz R, Huttner H, *et al.* Resistive-polymer versus forced-air warming: comparable efficacy in orthopedic patients. *Anesth Analg* 2010; **110**: 834–838.

300. Roth JV. Warming blankets should not be placed over transdermal medications. *Anesth Analg* 2002; **94**: 1043.

301. Negishi C, Hasegawa K, Mukai S, *et al.* Resistive-heating and forced-air warming

are comparably effective. *Anesth Analg* 2003; **96**: 1683–1687.

302. Matsuzaki Y, Matsukawa T, Ohki K, *et al.* Warming by resistive heating maintains perioperative normothermia as well as forced air heating. *Br J Anaesth* 2003; **90**: 689–691.

303. Nesher N, Wolf T, Uretzky G, *et al.* A novel thermoregulatory system maintains perioperative normothermia in children undergoing elective surgery. *Pediatr Anesth* 2001; **11**: 555–560.

304. Janicki PK, Higgins MS, Janssen J, Johnson RF and Beattie C. Comparison of two different temperature maintainance strategies during open abdominal surgery: upper body forced-air warming versus whole body water garment. *Anesthesiology* 2001; **95**: 868–874.

305. Bräuer A, Pacholik L, Perl T, *et al.* Wärmetransfer bei konduktiver Wärmung durch Wassermatten. *Anasthesiol Intensivmed Notfallmed Schmerzther* 2004; **39**: 471–476.

306. Perl T, Flöther L, Weyland W, Quintel M and Bräuer A. Comparison of forced-air warming and resistive heating. *Minerva Anestesiol* 2008; **74**: 687–690.

307. Röder G, Sessler DI, Roth G, *et al.* Intra-operative rewarming with Hot Dog® resistive heating and forced-air heating: a trial of lower-body warming. *Anaesthesia* 2011; **66**: 667–674.

308. Egan C, Bernstein E, Reddy D, *et al.* A randomized comparison of intraoperative PerfecTemp and forced-air warming during open abdominal surgery. *Anesth Analg* 2011; **113**: 1076–1081.

309. Brandes IF, Müller C, Perl T, *et al.* Effektivität einer neuen Wärmedecke. Eine prospektiv randomisierte Studie [Efficacy of a novel warming blanket: prospective randomized trial]. *Anaesthesist* 2013; **62**: 137–142.

310. Leung KK, Lai A and Wu A. A randomised controlled trial of the electric heating pad vs forced-air warming for preventing hypothermia during laparotomy. *Anaesthesia* 2007; **62**: 605–608.

311. Kimberger O, Held C, Stadelmann K, *et al.* Resistive polymer versus forced-air warming: comparable heat transfer and core rewarming rates in volunteers. *Anesth Analg* 2008; **107**: 1621–1626.

312. De Witte JL, Demeyer C and Vandemaele E. Resistive-heating or forced-air warming for the prevention of redistribution hypothermia. *Anesth Analg* 2010; **110**: 829–833.

313. Perez-Protto S, Sessler DI, Reynolds LF, *et al.* Circulating-water garment or the combination of a circulating-water mattress and forced-air cover to maintain core temperature during major upper-abdominal surgery. *Br J Anaesth* 2010; **105**: 466–470.

314. Hasegawa K, Negishi C, Nakagawa F and Ozaki M. Core temperatures during major abdominal surgery in patients warmed with new circulating-water garment, forced-air warming, or carbon-fiber resistive-heating system. *J Anesth* 2012; **26**: 168–173.

315. Sury MR and Scuplak S. Water-filled garment warming of infants undergoing open abdominal or thoracic surgery. *Pediatr Surg Int* 2006; **22**: 182–185.

316. Galvao CM, Liang Y and Clark AM. Effectiveness of cutaneous warming systems on temperature control: meta-analysis. *J Adv Nurs* 2010; **66**: 1196–1206.

317. Bräuer A, Zink W, Timmermann A, Perl T and Quintel M. Strategien zur Vermeidung von perioperativer Hypothermie bei Off-Pump-Bypass-Chirurgie. *Anästh Intensivmed* 2011; **52**: 251–262.

318. Wong PF, Kumar S, Bohra A, Whetter D and Leaper DJ. Randomized clinical trial of perioperative systemic warming in major elective abdominal surgery. *Br J Surg* 2007; **94**: 421–426.

319. Henriques FC and Moritz AR. Studies of thermal injury. I.The conduction of heat to and through skin and the temperatures attained herein.A theoretitcal and an experimental investigation. *Am J Pathol* 1947; **23**: 531–549.

320. Moritz AR and Henriques FC. Studies of thermal injury. II. The relative importance of time and surface temperature in the causation of cutaneous burns. *Am J Pathol* 1947: 695–720.

321. Crino MH and Nagel EL. Thermal burns by warming blankets in the operation room. *Anesthesiology* 1968; **29**: 149–150.

322. Sadove RC and Furgasen TG. Major thermal burn as a result of intraoperative heating blanket use. *J Burn Care Rehabil* 1992; **13**: 443–445.

323. Dewar DJ, Fraser JF, Choo KL and Kimble RM. Thermal injuries in three children caused by an electrical warming mattress. *Br J Anaesth* 2004; **93**: 586–589.

324. Acikel C, Kale B and Celikoz B. Major thermal burn due to intraoperative heating blanket malfunction. *Burns* 2002; **28**: 283–284.

325. Gali B, Findlay jY and Plevak DJ. Skin injury with the use of a water warming device. *Anesthesiology* 2003; **98**: 1509–1510.

326. Clarke PA and Thornton MJ. Failure of a water-bath design intravenous fluid warmer. *Can J Anaesth* 2009; **56**: 876–877.

327. Schmidt JH, Weyland W, Fritz U, *et al.* Experimentelle Untersuchung zur Effektivitat verschiedener Infusions- und Blutwärmeverfahren. *Anaesthesist* 1996; **45**: 1067–1074.

328. Moerer O, Bräuer A, Weyland W and Braun U. Erwärmungseffektivität und Erythrozytentraumatisierung verschiedener Infusions- und Bluterwärmungssysteme. *Anasthesiol Intensivmed Notfallmed Schmerzther* 2004; **39**: 138–146.

329. Burns S. An investigation of surgical infections reveals a fluid warmer as a reservoir for bacteria. *Am J Infect Control* 1999; **27**: 216.

330. Andrzejowski JC, Turnbull D, Nandakumar A, Gowthaman S and Eapen G. A randomised single blinded study of the administration of pre-warmed fluid vs active fluid warming on the incidence of peri-operative hypothermia in short surgical procedures. *Anaesthesia* 2010; **65**: 942–945.

331. [No authors listed] In-line blood/solution warmers. *Health Devices* 1996; **25**: 352–388.

332. Horowitz PE, Delagarza MA, Pulaski JJ and Smith RA. Flow rates and warming efficacy with Hotline and Ranger blood/fluid warmers. *Anesth Analg* 2004; **99**: 788–792.

333. Comunale ME. A laboratory evaluation of the Level 1 Rapid Infuser (H1025) and the Belmont Instrument Fluid Management System (FMS 2000) for rapid transfusion. *Anesth Analg* 2003; **97**: 1064–1069.

334. Campbell G, Alderson P, Smith AF and Warttig S. Warming of intravenous and irrigation fluids for preventing inadvertent perioperative hypothermia. *Cochrane Database Syst Rev* 2015; **4**: CD009891.

335. Camus Y, Delva E, Cohen S and Lienhart A. The effects of warming intravenous fluids on intraoperative hypothermia and postoperative shivering during prolonged abdominal surgery. *Acta Anaesthesiol Scand* 1996; **40**: 779–782.

336. Sieunarine K and White GH. Full-thickness burn and venous thrombosis following intravenous infusion of microwave-heated crystalloid fluids. *Burns* 1996; **22**: 568–569.

337. Husser CS, Chamblee B, Brown MJ, Long TR and Wass CT. Inductive warming of intravenous fluids: overheating of the toroid heating element during rapid infusion. *Anesthesiology* 2004; **101**: 1019–1021.

338. Arrandale L and Ng L. Superficial burn caused by a Hotline fluid warmer infusion set. *Anaesthesia* 2009; **64**: 101–102.

339. Wilson S and Szerb J. Failure of an iv fluid warming device. *Can J Anesth* 2007; **54**: 324–325.

340. Jin Y, Tian J, Sun M and Yang K. A systematic review of randomised controlled trials of the effects of warmed irrigation fluid on core body temperature during endoscopic surgeries. *J Clin Nurs* 2011; **20**: 305–316.

341. Jo YY, Chang YJ, Kim YB, Lee S and Kwak HJ. Effect of preoperative forced-air warming on hypothermia in elderly

patients undergoing transurethral resection of the prostate. *Urol J* 2015; **12**: 2366–2370.

342. Jaffe JS, McCullough C, Harkaway RC and Ginsberg PC. Effects of irrigation fluid temperature on core body temperature during transurethral resection of the prostate. *Urology* 2001; **57**: 1078–1081.

343. Pan X, Ye L, Liu Z, *et al.* Effect of irrigation fluid temperature on core body temperature and inflammatory response during arthroscopic shoulder surgery. *Arch Orthop Trauma Surg* 2015; **135**: 1131–1139.

344. Bräuer A, Perl T, Uyanik Z, *et al.* Perioperative thermal insulation: only little clinically important differences? *Br J Anaesth* 2004; **92**: 836–840.

345. Kaufman WC, Bothe D and Meyer SD. Thermal insulating capabilities of outdoor clothing materials. *Science* 1982; **215**: 690–691.

346. Sessler DI, McGuire J and Sessler AM. Perioperative thermal insulation. *Anesthesiology* 1991; **74**: 875–879.

347. Maglinger PE, Sessler DI and Lenhardt R. Cutaneous heat loss with three surgical drapes, one impervious to moisture. *Anesth Analg* 2005; **100**: 738–742.

348. Bräuer A, Perl T, English MJ and Quintel M. Perioperative thermal insulation. *Surg Technol Int* 2007; **16**: 41–45.

349. Hirvonen EA and Niskanen M. Thermal suits as an alternative way to keep patients warm peri-operatively: a randomised trial. *Eur J Anaesthesiol* 2011; **28**: 376–381.

350. Rathinam S, Annam V, Steyn R and Raghuraman G. A randomised controlled trial comparing Mediwrap heat retention and forced air warming for maintaining normothermia in thoracic surgery. *Interact CardioVasc Thorac Surg* 2009; **9**: 15–19.

351. Leben J, Kurz-Müller K and Tryba M. Warming devices in pediatric anesthesia. *Ann N Y Acad Sci* 1997; **813**: 812–817.

352. Bennett J, Ramachandra V, Webster J and Carli F. Prevention of hypothermia during hip surgery: effect of passive compared with active skin surface warming. *Br J Anaesth* 1994; **73**: 180–183.

353. Berti M, Casati A, Torri G, *et al.* Active warming, not passive heat retention, maintains normothermia during combined epidural-general anesthesia for hip and knee arthroplasty. *J Clin Anesth* 1997; **9**: 482–486.

354. Simmons M, Phillips P, Doctor U and Liehr P. The effect of two intraoperative heat-conserving methods on orthopedic patients receiving regional and general anesthesia. *J Post Anesth Nurs* 1992; **7**: 170–175.

355. Alderson P, Campbell G, Smith AF, *et al.* Thermal insulation for preventing inadvertent perioperative hypothermia. *Cochrane Database Syst Rev* 2014; **6**: CD009908.

356. Torrie JJ, Yip P and Robinson E. Comparison of forced-air warming and radiant heating during transurethral prostatic resection under spinal anaesthesia. *Anaesth Intensive Care* 2005; **33**: 733–738.

357. Weyland W, Weyland A, Hellige G, *et al.* Efficiency of a new radiant heater for postoperative rewarming. *Acta Anaesthesiol Scand* 1994; **38**: 601–606.

358. Henneberg S, Eklund A, Joachimsson PO, Stjernström H and Wiklund L. Effects of a thermal ceiling on postoperative hypothermia. *Acta Anaesthesiol Scand* 1985; **29**: 602–606.

359. Eckerbom B and Lindholm C-E. Heat and moisture exchangers and the body temperature: a peroperative study. *Acta Anaesthesiol Scand* 1990; **34**: 538–542.

360. Goldberg ME, Epstein R, Rosenblum F, *et al.* Do heated humidifiers and heat and moisture exchangers prevent temperature drop during lower abdominal surgery? *J Clin Anesth* 1992; **4**: 16–20.

361. Kulkarni P, Webster J and Carli F. Body heat transfer during hip surgery using active core warming. *Can J Anaesth* 1995; **42**: 571–576.

362. Bissonnette B and Sessler DI. Passive or active inspired gas humidification increases thermal steady-state

temperatures in anesthetized infants. *Anesth Analg* 1989; **69**: 783–787.

363. Kim E, Lee SY, Lim YJ, *et al.* Effect of a new heated and humidified breathing circuit with a fluid-warming device on intraoperative core temperature: a prospective randomized study. *J Anesth* 2015; **29**: 499–507.

364. Bräuer A and Weyland W. Oesophageal heat exchanger in the prevention of perioperative hypothermia. *Acta Anaesthesiol Scand* 1998; **42**: 1232–1233.

365. Kristensen G, Guldager H and Gravesen H. Prevention of peroperative hypothermia in abdominal surgery. *Acta Anaesthesiol Scand* 1986; **30**: 314–316.

366. Rasmussen YH, Leikersfeldt G and Drenck NE. Forced-air surface warming versus oesophageal heat exchanger in the prevention of peroperative hypothermia. *Acta Anaesthesiol Scand* 1998; **42**: 348–352.

367. Grahn D, Brock-Utne JG, Watenpaugh DE and Heller HC. Recovery from mild hypothermia can be accelerated by mechanically distending blood vessels in the hand. *J Appl Physiol (1985)* 1998; **85**: 1643–1648.

368. Ruetzler K, Kovaci B, Guloglu E, *et al.* Forced-air and a novel patient-warming system (vitalHEAT vH2) comparably maintain normothermia during open abdominal surgery. *Anesth Analg* 2011; **112**: 608–614.

369. Plattner O, Ikeda T, Sessler DI, Christensen R and Turakhia M. Postanesthetic vasoconstriction slows peripheral-to-core transfer of cutaneous heat, thereby isolating the core thermal compartment. *Anesth Analg* 1997; **85**: 899–906.

370. Smith CE, Parand A, Pinchak AC, Hagen JF and Hancock DE. The failure of negative pressure rewarming (Thermostat™) to accelate recovery from mild hypothermia in postoperative surgical patients. *Anesth Analg* 1999; **89**: 1541–1545.

371. Prunet B, Asencio Y, Lacroix G, *et al.* Maintenance of normothermia during burn surgery with an intravascular temperature control system: a non-randomised controlled trial. *Injury* 2012; **43**: 648–652.

372. Taylor EE, Carroll JP, Lovitt MA, *et al.* Active intravascular rewarming for hypothermia associated with traumatic injury: early experience with a new technique. *Proc (Bayl Univ Med Cent)* 2008; **21**: 120–126.

373. Prunet B, Lacroix G, Bordes J, *et al.* Catheter related venous thrombosis with cooling and warming catheters: two case reports. *Cases J* 2009; **2**: 8857.

374. Selldén E, Bränström R and Brundin T. Preoperative infusion of amino acids prevents postoperative hypothermia. *Br J Anaesth* 1996; **76**: 227–234.

375. Selldén E and Lindahl SGE. Amino acid-induced thermogenesis to prevent hypothermia during anesthesia is not associated with increased stress response. *Anesth Analg* 1998; **87**: 637–640.

376. Kasai T, Nakajima Y, Matsukawa T, *et al.* Effect of preoperative amino acid infusion on thermoregulatory response during spinal anaesthesia. *Br J Anaesth* 2003; **90**: 58–61.

377. Widman J, Hammarqvist F and Selldén E. Amino acid infusion induces thermogenesis and reduces blood loss during hip arthroplasty under spinal anesthesia. *Anesth Analg* 2002; **95**: 1757–1762.

378. Inoue S, Shinjo T, Kawaguchi M, Nakajima Y and Furuya H. Amino acid infusions started after development of intraoperative core hypothermia do not affect rewarming but reduce the incidence of postoperative shivering during major abdominal surgery: a randomized trial. *J Anesth* 2011; **25**: 850–854.

379. Mizobe T, Nakajima Y, Ueno H and Sessler DI. Fructose administration increases intraoperative core temperature by augmenting both metabolic rate and the vasoconstriction threshold. *Anesthesiology* 2006; **104**: 1124–1130.

380. Coburn M, Rossaint R, Bause H, *et al.* Qualitätsindikatoren Anästhesiologie

2015. *Anästh Intensivmed* 2016; **57**: 219–230.

381. Menzel M, Grote R, Leuchtmann D, et al. Implementation of a thermal management concept to prevent perioperative hypothermia: results of a 6 month period in clinical practice. *Anaesthesist* 2016; **65**: 423–429.

382. Bräuer A, Brandes IF, Perl T, Wetz AJ and Bauer M. Vorwärmung: Von der Kür zur Pflicht. [Prewarming: Yesterday's luxury, today's minimum requirement]. *Anaesthesist* 2014; **63**: 406–414.

383. Hynson JM, Sessler DI, Moayeri A, McGuire J and Schroeder M. The effects of preinduction warming on temperature and blood pressure during propofol/nitrous oxide anesthesia. *Anesthesiology* 1993; **79**: 219–228, discussion.

384. Bräuer A, Waeschle RM, Heise D, et al. Präoperative Vorwärmung in der klinischen Routine: Erste Erfahrungen. [Preoperative prewarming as a routine measure: First experiences]. *Anaesthesist* 2010; **59**: 842–850.

385. Fossum S, Hays J and Henson MM. A comparison study on the effects of prewarming patients in the outpatient surgery setting. *J Perianesth Nurs* 2001; **16**: 187–194.

386. Horn E-P, Schroeder F, Gottschalk A, et al. Active warming during cesarean delivery. *Anesth Analg* 2002; **94**: 409–414.

387. Chung SH, Lee BS, Yang HJ, et al. Effect of preoperative warming during cesarean section under spinal anesthesia. *Korean J Anesthesiol* 2012; **62**: 454–460.

388. de Brito Poveda V, Clark AM and Galvao CM. A systematic review on the effectiveness of prewarming to prevent perioperative hypothermia. *J Clin Nurs* 2013; **22**: 906–918.

389. Roberson MC, Dieckmann LS, Rodriguez RE and Austin PN. A review of the evidence for active preoperative warming of adults undergoing general anesthesia. *AANA J* 2013; **81**: 351–356.

390. Vanni SMD, Castiglia YMM, Ganem EM, et al. Preoperative warming combined with intraoperative skin-surface warming does not avoid hypothermia caused by spinal anesthesia in patients with midazolam premedication. *Sao Paulo Med J* 2007; **125**: 144–149.

391. O'Brien D, Greenfield ML, Anderson JE, Smith BA and Morris M. Comfort, satisfaction, and anxiolysis in surgical patients using a patient-adjustable comfort warming system: a prospective randomized clinical trial. *J Perianesth Nurs* 2010; **25**: 88–93.

392. Brandes IF, Jipp M, Popov AF, et al. Intensified thermal management for patients undergoing transcatheter aortic valve implantation (TAVI). *J Cardiothorac Surg* 2011; **6**: 117.

393. Machata AM, Willschke H, Kabon B, Prayer D and Marhofer P. Effect of brain magnetic resonance imaging on body core temperature in sedated infants and children. *Br J Anaesth* 2009; **102**: 385–389.

394. Lipsett PA. Do we really need laminar flow ventilation in the operating room to prevent surgical site infections? *Ann Surg* 2008; **248**: 701–703.

395. Tumia N and Ashcroft GP. Convection warmers: a possible source of contamination in laminar airflow operating theatres? *J Hosp Infect* 2002; **52**: 171–174.

396. Todd MM, Hindman BJ, Clarke WR and Torner JC for the Intraoperative Hypothermia for Aneurysm Surgery Trial (IHAST) Investigators. Mild intraoperative hypothermia during surgery for intracranial aneurysm. *N Engl J Med* 2005; **352**: 135–145.

397. Jung KT, Kim SH, Lee HY, et al. Effect on thermoregulatory responses in patients undergoing a tympanoplasty in accordance to the anesthetic techniques during PEEP: a comparison between inhalation anesthesia with desflurane and TIVA. *Korean J Anesthesiol* 2014; **67**: 32–37.

398. Sumer BD, Myers LL, Leach J and Truelson JM. Correlation between intraoperative hypothermia and perioperative morbidity in patients with

head and neck cancer. *Arch Otolaryngol Head Neck Surg* 2009; **135**: 682–686.

399. Chiang S, Cohen B and Blackwell K. Myocardial infarction after microvascular head and neck reconstruction. *Laryngoscope* 2002; **112**: 1849–1852.

400. Cywinski JB, Xu M, Sessler DI, Mason D and Koch CG. Predictors of prolonged postoperative endotracheal intubation in patients undergoing thoracotomy for lung resection. *J Cardiothorac Vasc Anesth* 2009; **23**: 766–769.

401. Mäkinen M-T. Comparison of body temperature changes during laparoscopic and open cholecystectomy. *Acta Anaesthesiol Scand* 1997; **41**: 736–740.

402. Danelli G, Berti M, Perotti V, *et al.* Temperature control and recovery of bowel function after laparoscopic or laparotomic colorectal surgery in patients receiving combined epidural/general anesthesia and postoperative epidural analgesia. *Anesth Analg* 2002; **95**: 467–71, table.

403. Luck AJ, Moyes D, Maddern GJ and Hewett PJ. Core temperature changes during open and laparoscopic colorectal surgery. *Surg Endosc* 1999; **13**: 480–483.

404. Sultan P, Habib AS, Cho Y and Carvalho B. The effect of patient warming during caesarean delivery on maternal and neonatal outcomes: a meta-analysis. *Br J Anaesth* 2015; **115**: 500–510.

405. Horn EP, Bein B, Steinfath M, *et al.* The incidence and prevention of hypothermia in newborn bonding after cesarean delivery: a randomized controlled trial. *Anesth Analg* 2014; **118**: 997–1002.

406. Butwick AJ, Lipman SS and Carvalho B. Intraoperative forced air-warming during cesarean delivery under spinal anesthesia does not prevent maternal hypothermia. *Anesth Analg* 2007; **105**: 1413–1419.

407. Cobb B, Cho Y, Hilton G, Ting V and Carvalho B. Active warming utilizing combined IV fluid and forced-air warming decreases hypothermia and improves maternal comfort during cesarean delivery: a randomized control trial. *Anesth Analg* 2016; **122**: 1490–1497.

408. Perlman J and Kjaer K. Neonatal and maternal temperature regulation during and after delivery. *Anesth Analg* 2016; **123**: 168–172.

409. Görges M, Ansermino JM and Whyte SD. A retrospective audit to examine the effectiveness of preoperative warming on hypothermia in spine deformity surgery patients. *Paediatr Anaesth* 2013; **23**: 1054–1061.

410. Sessler DI. Forced-air warming in infants and children. *Paediatr Anaesth* 2013; **23**: 467–468.

411. Pearce B, Christensen R and Voelpel-Lewis T. Perioperative hypothermia in the pediatric population: prevalence, risk factors and outcomes. *J Anesth Clin Res* 2010; **1**: 102.

412. Morehouse D, Williams L, Lloyd C, *et al.* Perioperative hypothermia in NICU infants: its occurrence and impact on infant outcomes. *Adv Neonatal Care* 2014; **14**: 154–164.

413. Donnino MW, Andersen LW, Berg KM, *et al.* Temperature management after cardiac arrest: an advisory statement by the Advanced Life Support Task Force of the International Liaison Committee on Resuscitation and the American Heart Association Emergency Cardiovascular Care Committee and the Council on Cardiopulmonary, Critical Care, Perioperative and Resuscitation. *Resuscitation* 2016; **98**: 97–104.

414. Merchant RM, Abella BS, Peberdy MA, *et al.* Therapeutic hypothermia after cardiac arrest: unintentional overcooling is common using ice packs and conventional cooling blankets. *Crit Care Med* 2006; **34**: S490–S494.

415. Bro-Jeppesen J, Hassager C, Wanscher M, *et al.* Post-hypothermia fever is associated with increased mortality after out-of-hospital cardiac arrest. *Resuscitation* 2013; **84**: 1734–1740.

416. Warttig S, Alderson P, Campbell G and Smith AF. Interventions for treating inadvertent postoperative hypothermia. *Cochrane Database Syst Rev* 2014; **11**: CD009892.

417. Lennon RL, Hosking MP, Conover MA and Perkins WJ. Evaluation of a forced-air system for warming hypothermic postoperative patients. *Anesth Analg* 1990; **70**: 424–427.

418. Alfonsi P, Nourredine KEA, Adam F, Chauvin M and Sessler DI. Effect of postoperative skin-surface warming on oxygen consumption and the shivering threshold. *Anaesthesia* 2003; **58**: 1228–1234.

419. Weyland W, Fritz U, Fabian S, *et al.* [Postoperative warming therapy in the recovery room: a comparison of radiative and convective warmers] Postoperative Warmetherapie im Aufwachraum: Ein Vergleich von radiativer und konvektiver Warmezufuhr. *Anaesthesist* 1994; **43**: 648–657.

420. Alfonsi P, Sessler DI, Du Manoir B, *et al.* The effects of meperidine and sufentanil on the shivering threshold in postoperative patients. *Anesthesiology* 1998; **89**: 43–48.

421. Alfonsi P, Passard A, Gaude-Joindreau V, *et al.* Nefopam and alfentanil additively reduce the shivering threshold in humans whereas nefopam and clonidine do not. *Anesthesiology* 2009; **111**: 102–109.

422. Wrench IJ, Singh P, Dennis AR, Mahajan RP and Crossley AWA. The minimum effective doses of pethidine and doxapram in the treatment of post-anaesthetic shivering. *Anaesthesia* 1997; **52**: 32–36.

423. Horn E-P, Standl T, Sessler DI *et al.* Physostigmine prevents postanesthetic shivering as does Meperidine or Clonidine. *Anesthesiology* 1998; **88**: 108–113.

424. Mokhtarani M, Mahgoub AN, Morioka N *et al.* Buspirone and meperidine synergistically reduce the shivering threshold. *Anesth Analg* 2001; **93**: 1233–1239.

425. Alfonsi P, Adam F, Passard A, *et al.* Nefopam, a nonsedative benzoxazocine analgesic, selectively reduces the shivering threshold in unanesthetized subjects. *Anesthesiology* 2004; **100**: 37–43.

426. Delaunay L, Bonnet F, Liu N, *et al.* Clonidine comparably decreases the thermoregulatory thresholds for vasoconstriction and shivering in humans. *Anesthesiology* 1993; **79**: 470–474.

427. Lewis SR, Nicholson A, Smith AF and Alderson P. Alpha-2 adrenergic agonists for the prevention of shivering following general anaesthesia. *Cochrane Database Syst Rev* 2015; **8**: CD011107.

428. Joris J, Banache M, Bonnet F, Sessler DI and Lamy M. Clonidine and ketanserin both are effective treatment for postanesthetic shivering. *Anesthesiology* 1993; **79**: 532–539.

429. Callaway CW, Elmer J, Guyette FX *et al.* Dexmedetomidine reduces shivering during mild hypothermia in waking subjects. *PLoS One* 2015; **10**: e0129709.

430. Fritz HG, Hoff H, Hartmann M, Karzai W and Schwarzkopf KR. The effects of urapidil on thermoregulatory thresholds in volunteers. *Anesth Analg* 2001; **94**: 626–630.

431. Lenhardt R, Orhan-Sungur M, Komatsu R *et al.* Suppression of shivering during hypothermia using a novel drug combination in healthy volunteers. *Anesthesiology* 2009; **111**: 110–115.

432. Kose EA, Dal D, Akinci SB, Saricaoglu F and Aypar U. The efficacy of ketamine for the treatment of postoperative shivering. *Anesth Analg* 2008; **106**: 120–122.

433. Tie HT, Su GZ, He K, *et al.* Efficacy and safety of ondansetron in preventing postanesthesia shivering: a meta-analysis of randomized controlled trials. *BMC Anesthesiol* 2014; **14**: 12.

434. Kranke P, Eberhart LH, Roewer N and Tramer MR. Pharmacological treatment of postoperative shivering: a quantitative systematic review of randomized controlled trials. *Anesth Analg* 2002; **94**: 453–460.

Index

accidental hypothermia, 26
activated partial
    thromboplastin time, 88
active rewarming, 169, 184–
    185
adhesive water mattresses,
    143–144
airway, 32
airway heating and
    humidification, 164
alfentanil, 50, 185
amino acids, 167
amplification phase of
    coagulation, 85
angiogenesis, 104
anorexia nervosa, 33
antidepressant, 35
antipsychotic, 36
arrhythmia, 3, 94, 98, 100
arteriovenous shunt, 21, 23,
    53, 59
arthroscopic surgery, 158
atracurium, 83
atropine, 38, 40
autonomic thermoregulation,
    9, 16, 18, 20, 36, 44
axillary temperature, 127
Aδ-fibre, 13, 61

behavioural thermoregulation,
    15, 17–18, 44
benzodiazepine, 37, 53, 65
bladder temperature, 124
blood loss, 85, 89
brown adipose tissue, 25
buspirone, 186

caesarean section, 107, 181
carbon dioxide production, 26
cardiac arrest, 3, 98, 100
C-fibre, 13, 61
chemotaxis, 103–104
circadian rhythm, 17
circulating water mattress, 5,
    143
clonidine, 38–39, 66, 186
clot formation time, 88
clotting time, 88
cold-sensitive neuron, 19

conduction, 29, 31, 55
conductive warmer, 5, 143,
    169, 180
    pressure ulcer, 150
    risk of burns, 147
convection, 29–30, 55
core temperature, 17, 33,
    115
costs, 103, 109
cytochrome P450, 78–79

desflurane, 48, 79
dexmedetomidine, 65, 66,
    186
diabetes mellitus, 33
distal oesophagus, 116–117
dolasetron, 39
double-sensor thermometer,
    114, 124

EEG, 80, 142
emissivity, 28
endovascular warming
    catheter, 166
energy expenditure, 26–27, 66
enflurane, 46, 79
ENT surgery, 48, 180
ephedrine, 55
epidural anaesthesia, 59, 63, 68
evaporation, 31–32, 55, 73

feeling cold, 91
fever, 26, 93
fluid warmer, 3, 5, 152, 179
    air embolism, 157
    risk of burns, 156
    risk of infection, 156
flunitrazepam, 38
forced-air warmer, 5, 29, 128,
    169, 178
    laminar air flow, 139, 141
    noise, 142
    overheating, 138
    risk of burns, 138
forearm–fingertip temperature
    gradient, 22, 93
fructose, 167

guideline, 8, 72, 155, 168

halothane, 45–46, 79
heat- and moisture-
    exchanging filters
    (HME), 164
heat balance, 32
heat exchange, 9
heat loss, 8, 32, 52, 55, 59–60,
    68
heat loss from surgical
    incision, 73
heat production, 44
heat production of the body,
    32, 52, 55, 59
hereditary fructose
    intolerance, 167
hyperthermia, 26
hypothalamus, 10, 15–16, 18,
    22, 25, 46, 61
hypothyreosis, 35
hypoxaemia, 94, 96

iliac artery, 116
incidence of perioperative
    hypothermia, 75
infrared thermometry of the
    aural canal, 126
infrared-A, 162
infrared-B, 162
infrared-C, 162
infrared-thermometer, 111
initiation phase, 85
insula, 15–17
insulation, 159, 161, 180
interferon-γ, 104
interleukin-2 (IL-2), 104
intra-abdominal surgery, 180
intracerebral surgery, 180
irrigation fluid, 74, 158
isoflurane, 47, 79

ketamine, 65–66, 186

lateral spinothalamic tract,
    14–16
length of stay
    hospital stay, 109
    intensive care unit, 109
    postanaesthetic care unit, 97
leukocyte, 104

limbic system, 15–16
linear phase, 52, 55
lymphocyte, 104

malignant hyperthermia, 26, 115
mass insulator, 159, 161
massive transfusion, 3
maximum clot firmness, 88
meperidine, 50, 185–186
midazolam, 37–39, 50, 65–66, 80
mivacurium, 84
morphine, 63
muscle relaxants, 52, 81
myocardial infarction, 98, 100, 102
myocardial ischaemia, 94, 98, 100

nasopharynx, 116, 121
nefopam, 185
negative pressure warmer, 165
neostigmine, 84
neuraxial anaesthesia, 59, 61–62, 172
newborns, 4, 25, 55, 181
non-shivering thermogenesis, 25
non-thermoregulatory shivering, 92–93

obesity, 32, 54–55
oesophageal warmer, 165
ondansetron, 39, 186
operating room temperature, 71
opioids, 40, 50, 65, 81
oral temperature, 123
orthopaedic surgery, 89, 96, 107, 181
oxidative killing, 104
oxygen consumption, 26

paediatric surgery, 183
pain, 93–94, 96
paraplegia, 35
patients undergoing targeted temperature management, 183
peripheral nerve block, 64
phagocytosis, 104
pharmacodynamics, 80
pharmacokinetics, 78–79, 81

phenylephrine, 55, 62
plasmatic coagulation, 85–86
plateau phase, 52, 55
platelet function, 85–86, 88
pneumonia, 107
postoperative protein catabolism, 108
premedication, 36
prewarming, 62, 168–170
  induction room, 172
  on the ward, 172
  preoperative holding area, 172
prilocain, 84
propagation phase, 85
propofol, 49, 65, 80
prothrombin time, 88
pulmonary artery, 116

radiant insulator, 159, 161
radiation, 28, 30, 55
radiative warmer, 162
rectal temperature, 125
redistribution of heat, 44, 52, 54–55, 59, 62, 68, 170, 172
redistribution phase, 52, 54
regional anaesthesia, 59, 65–66
remifentanil, 50, 65–66, 81, 93
rocuronium, 81, 83
rotational thrombelastometry, 88

sedation, 65
self-warming blankets, 144
sepsis, 107
sevoflurane, 48, 79
shivering, 5, 16, 21, 23, 52, 60, 91, 92, 94
  oxygen uptake, 8, 93
  thermoregulatory shivering, 23
spinal anaesthesia, 59, 63, 66
subcutaneous tissue oxygenation, 103
sublingual temperature, 123
sugammadex, 84
surgical skin preparation, 72–73
sweating, 16, 21, 31

temperature-sensitive neuron, 10
temporal artery temperature, 127

tetraplegia, 35
thalamus, 10, 15
thermal steady state, 17, 170
thermistor, 111
thermocouple, 111
thermoreceptor, 9–11
thermoregulation, 8–9, 44, 59, 61
thermoregulatory shivering, 92–93
thermoregulatory threshold, 44
thermoregulatory vasoconstriction, 21, 32, 103
thermosensation, 9–10
thermosensitive neuron, 12, 16, 19
thoracic surgery, 180
thrombelastography, 88
tourniquet, 56
tramadol, 185
transfusion requirement, 85, 89
transurethral resection of the prostate, 74, 158
treatment of shivering, 184–185
TRP channel, 10–11
tumour necrosis factor-α (TNF-α), 104
tympanic membrane, 113, 116, 119

unstable angina, 98, 100
urapidil, 186

vasoconstriction, 16, 21
vasodilation, 16, 21
vecuronium, 81
von Willebrand Factor (vWF), 85

warm-sensitive neuron, 19–20, 46
water warming garment, 143–144
wound infection, 103, 105, 107
wound infections, 105
wound temperature, 88–89

zero-heat-flux thermometer, 111, 113, 124

Printed in the United States
by Baker & Taylor Publisher Services

Printed in the United States
by Baker & Taylor Publisher Services